Working with Bereaved People

Ann Faulkner MA PhD MLitt DipEd SRN RCNT

Professor of Communication Skills in Health Care, Medical School, University of Sheffield, Sheffield, UK

Deputy Director, Trent Palliative Care Centre, Sheffield, UK

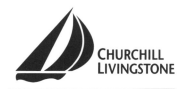

CHURCHILL
LIVINGSTONE

EDINBURGH HONG KONG LONDON MADRID MELBOURNE
NEW YORK AND TOKYO 1995

CHURCHILL LIVINGSTONE
An imprint of Harcourt Brace and Company Limited

© Pearson Professional Limited 1995
© Harcourt Brace and Company Limited 1998

⬙ is a registered trademark of Harcourt Brace and
Company Limited

First published 1995
    Reprinted 1996
    Reprinted 1998

ISBN 0 443 051445

British Library of Cataloguing in Publication Data
A catalogue record for this book is available from the British Library.

Library of Congress Cataloging in Publication Data
A catalogue record for this book is available from the Library of Congress

The
publisher's
policy is to use
**paper manufactured
from sustainable forests**

Produced by Addison Wesley Longman China Limited, Hong Kong
EPC /03

Contents

Preface

The aim of writing this book was to produce a practical guide for those who work with bereaved people. The readers may be nurses, counsellors, other professionals, or volunteers. For that reason, I have written in a very practical manner using case studies from my own experience, both in working with bereaved people, but also in working with groups of students who want to know more about bereavement and who have shared their problem cases with me.

To make the book more readable, I have used the minimum of references and based most of the text on my own professional experience. However, I accept that many people will want to go further than the content of this book and to help to meet their needs, I have included a Further Reading List at the end of the book.

There is an increasing awareness of the needs of bereaved people. There is to date no government involvement in working with the bereaved, nor yet any national policy on how the needs of such people can be met. However, it is good to see change occurring. The organizations 'Cruse' and 'Help the Hospices' have recently combined to improve the training of bereavement counsellors, both within Cruse and from the hospice world. It is exciting to be working with that project and seeing the beginnings of a much more coherent course for those who work with the bereaved. To that end I hope this book will be of use.

I hope too that those who are not directly involved with bereavement work, but who care for the dying and their families, will find something of worth in the text. I make no apologies for the approach which is similar to the style in my previous work, *Effective Interaction with Patients* (Faulkner 1992).

Sheffield 1995   A.F.

Acknowledgements

This book would not have been written without the encouragement of professionals and volunteers, who have shared with me their problems in working with the bereaved. I hope that this book meets their expressed need for practical guidelines, and I thank them for continued positive feedback.

I would also like to thank Help the Hospices and the Extra-Mural Department of Manchester University, and others who have asked me to run workshops on working with the bereaved. I have learnt so much from these experiences.

My family have been ever supportive both at a practical level with endless tea and offers of help, and at an emotional level in their faith in my ability.

Last, but by no means least, I would like to thank Barbara Grimbley for typing the manuscript, correcting my errors and turning my scribbles into tables and figures.

1

The concept of loss

Bereavement temporarily sets an individual apart from friends and neighbours. It is not uncommon for those who have suffered a death in the family to describe how people who would normally stop and chat if they met in the street, would now cross the road rather than having to talk to them. Such behaviour is usually the result of embarrassment, and an inability to find the correct words to say to someone who has suffered the death of someone they love.

DISCOMFORT WITH DEATH

This discomfort with death and its aftermath may also apply to the health professionals who are expected to offer help and support at the time of death and subsequently. Simpson (1975) found that only 12% of nurses had experienced the death of a member of their own family before starting their training, and only 8% had seen a dead body. They may be apprehensive about discussing feelings both before and after a death, especially if they feel that they are ill-equipped for such a task.

The belief has therefore arisen that in order to understand and help a bereaved person one has to have had personal experience of death, and indeed in volunteer organizations, like Cruse, most of the counsellors are recruited after a suitable period of bereavement. Their motivation is to help others to cope with what they themselves found difficult.

VALUE AND LOSS

Death is a loss, and it is argued here that all members of the public and of the health professions learn to suffer loss from a very early age. It is this understanding of loss and its aftermath, no matter what the loss or how it was lost, that is the basis of understanding and having an empathetic response to the major loss of death.

Losses of childhood

Part of the socialization of a child from a very early age is to teach that child to put a value on both their own and other people's possessions. In the early years this is particularly true in terms of relationships, and it is not unusual to hear a small child talking about *my* mummy or *my* granny. It is well documented that when a second child arrives in a family the first child will need reassurance that the love that they take for granted will not change. Quite small children will feel so strongly about this that they check it out:

> Mary Ann was with her grandparents on the day that her sister was born. That evening, getting ready for bed, she suddenly spoke to her grandmother:
>
> Mary Ann: 'Granny, will you love the new baby?'
>
> Granny: 'Yes, of course I'll love the new baby'.
>
> Mary Ann: 'But you loved me first'.

Once a value has been put on a person or a possession, then subsequent loss is bound to bring grief. The level of that grief will be related to the importance of the loss. For example, a small child may have a lot of cuddly toys, but, in addition, a special toy that goes to bed with them every night, and in the car with them if they go on a strange journey. The child will react much more strongly if that toy is lost than if it were one that was a rare plaything and not a part of their lives. Melinda, for example, was heartbroken when she left her bedtime fluffy cat in a car that was subsequently stolen. The loss of the car meant little to the 2-year-old but she was inconsolable because her fluffy cat was not available at bedtime. This grief lasted for several days, and disrupted the child's sleep pattern.

The child's first loss of a person may be when friends move away and other friends have to come to take their place. The child will often mourn the fact that their best friend had to move and they will talk for a considerable time about where the friend is now, what are they doing and will ask if they will ever come back. If children themselves have to move, perhaps because their father gets a better job, then they experience loss both of the home that they had become accustomed to, and all their friends that they knew in the old house.

A child's first experience of death may be that of a pet. A favourite dog or cat may die or have an accident and the child will have to deal with their feelings about the death, about the burial, and about the aftermath. Hence, right from an early age a child gets used to the concept of loss, and gradually learns that nothing in the world is permanent. Such knowledge may never be verbalized nor explored, but the experience is there that will help them in the future to deal with more important losses.

Adolescent losses

As children move into adolescence, they begin to have their first major experiences in relationships. Few adolescents reach adulthood without the magic and the pain of first love. It is then that the young man or woman learns to invest their feelings in a person outside their immediate family circle. This is nowhere better epitomized than in Shakespeare's 'Romeo and Juliet', which demonstrates that the feelings for the other person may be so strong that they will transcend family values, family beliefs and family approval.

The sense of loss and rejection that follows the ending of the love affair make a deep and lasting impression. Such is the sense of desolation that some youngsters may feel very wary about ever loving again, although as they grow up these feelings lessen and most of them do invest in other relationships.

At the end of the first love affair, again the feelings might not be verbalized, but they include many of the features of grieving after a death (Ch. 4). They often include fantasies that the quarrel will be forgotten and that the loved one will return, even though the evidence is there to show that this is quite unlikely.

Adolescence is a time for other losses. School is a very

competitive environment, in terms of who gets into the hockey or the rugby team, who is top of the class, who gets to grammar school or who goes to private school, and then who goes on to University. For many children this is not important. They are happy with whatever space they have in life, but many are taught by their parents to be ambitious and to set certain goals, and if they are not met there is often a profound sense, not only of loss, but of failure and sometimes of rejection. All these emotions are possible, if amplified after the death of someone important in life.

Adult losses

Redundancy

In adulthood there are losses that are not as devastating as death but which, nevertheless, bring their own grief. When a coveted promotion does not happen or when a job is lost through redundancy, there is a sense of loss, and sometimes a questioning of one's own worth. There may be grief for some time following such an event and occasionally a sense of bitterness, too.

Divorce

The loss that is most akin to death is that of divorce, for very often it is one of the partners that leaves for a new love, and the other partner who is left desolate and feeling abandoned. Furthermore, they no longer have access to the loved person. This can lead to enormous feelings of frustration, anger and grief.

Jane had been married for 2 years to her childhood sweetheart when she realized that things were not as good between them as they had been. She went home to her mother on her days off to ask for advice, and subsequently decided to go home and talk frankly to her husband about her worries and concerns for the way things were between them.

Jane's husband was not expecting her home and when she arrived she found that he had another girl in their flat. He stated quite categorically that unless he could have the relationships that he wanted, he was no longer interested in staying married.

Jane moved out of the flat, feeling very unhappy, confused and almost in a state of disbelief. One day Jane rang her husband at work:

Husband: 'Why are you ringing me at work?'

Jane: 'There is something I want you to do'.

Husband: 'Oh, and what's that?'

Jane: 'I want you to go into the road and get run over by a bus'.

Jane was subsequently ashamed of her behaviour but she explained to a close friend that having a husband alive in the vicinity and yet unavailable to her was worse than if he were dead. Had he died, she would have been able to accept the fact that he was no longer available to her, or to anyone else.

MAGNITUDE OF LOSS

It is not possible to make assumptions about the magnitude of a loss whether it be of a possession, a pet, a person, or an ambition. From the examples in this chapter, the fluffy cat with which a small child slept was of far less magnitude in terms of loss than Jane's husband in divorce. However, at the time that the small child lost her fluffy cat, it may be that the intensity of loss was as great as for something that would have been accepted as more precious. What *is* different is that the cat could soon be replaced with another furry toy, though fond memories may remain of the original, whereas to replace Jane's husband with a new model would be impossible for a very long time.

Only the person suffering the loss can put a value on that loss, and it will be seen in subsequent chapters of this book that one of the vital roles of those working with bereaved people is to assess the magnitude of the loss from the individual's perspective.

CIRCUMSTANCES OF A LOSS

The circumstances of a loss can affect the way that an individual reacts to that loss. Some losses may be perceived as due to theft or carelessness.

Theft

Theft allows the person suffering the loss to blame someone else for what has happened. Jane blamed the new girlfriend for her husband's infidelity. Little Melinda blamed her father for the fact that her cat was lost in the car, and those who lose a coveted job or promotion may blame somebody else, either the person who took the job or the person who selected for the job.

These feelings give a natural focus for anger over the loss of something that was valued by the owner, or of a relationship that was valued by the person who feels rejected. This anger may be misdirected as often happens after a burglary when, rather than blaming those who have stolen treasured possessions, the police are blamed for not patrolling the area in a more effective way.

Carelessness

If the loss is perceived to be due to carelessness, then it brings with it a sense of guilt. When first love affairs break up, very often the rejected partner has a sense that somehow there was something they were not doing that caused the partner to reject them, and that the problems lie with themselves. They may feel that they are not beautiful enough to hold the lover's attention, or believe that they do not have the right background.

Similarly with divorce, very often the rejected partner feels that they did not come up to the expectations of their partner. Job losses may leave an individual with a sense of failure, and the loss of possessions may similarly carry with them a sense of guilt.

SOCIETY'S EXPECTATIONS

As people from childhood onwards try to make sense of their losses, no matter what their magnitude, there is often some confusion because of what is expected from them in the eyes of society.

Possessions

Possessions, for example, are seen to be readily replaceable.

Ann, at work, was describing a burglary and her friend interrupted and said:

Friend: 'But you were insured, weren't you?'

Ann: 'Yes, I was'.

Friend: 'Well then it doesn't matter'.

In fact it mattered enormously to Ann, because all her mother's jewellery had been stolen in the burglary. She did not wear it herself, but she had a fondness for it because it had belonged to her mother and she had planned to pass it on to her own daughters.

Pets

Similar attitudes may be taken with other, more serious, losses. When a pet dies there is often the comment that it is easy to get another puppy or kitten or whatever, so denying the undoubted affection that a family has for a pet that has been with them for a considerable time.

Stillbirth

Unfortunately, a very similar attitude is taken to those women who have a stillbirth. It seems to be forgotten that they have spent many months building a relationship with the unborn foetus within them and yet many have to face the comment,
'Well, you're young dear, you'll be able to have another'.
This 'easily replaceable' attitude to many losses can be reversed in the case of death. When somebody dies, they are often transformed into some sort of saint who was very much loved by everybody who knew them. This makes it incredibly difficult for someone who is bereaved, but who no longer cared for the person who died, to show their true feelings. People may be censured for not being sorry enough on the death of somebody who may have been very difficult during their lifetime.

LEARNING FROM LOSS

Those who work with bereaved people may themselves not have suffered bereavement in terms of the death of a loved one. However, most will have some losses in their own lives that will help them to empathize with those who have suffered the more major loss of death. To use those experiences of smaller losses requires that the individual has insight and develops some self-awareness of the way in which they coped with different losses. They also need to realize that different people cope in very different ways. Remembering previous important losses can aid empathetic responses to those who are bereaved.

Many adults have memories of early childhood losses and their reactions to those losses. For example, Molly at six had a black doll that was probably her favourite toy. Her mother had knitted various outfits for it and Molly spent many hours dressing and undressing her doll. Her elder brother, who liked to tease Molly, took the doll one day and hid it. Molly was desolate. She searched the house and could not find it. Finally her mother, in exasperation said,

'For goodness sake, just let's get ready for bed and when your brother comes in I'll ask him where it is'.

In fact, Molly's mother was busy and when her brother had come in she had forgotten to ask him where the doll was. Actually, he had hidden it in the flower bed in the garden. It was found in the morning after a storm, totally ruined, given that it was made of papier-mâché. Molly, as an adult, still remembers her sense of utter desolation and her scorn towards her parents who promised to buy her an identical doll.

The new doll sat in a corner of Molly's bedroom and was hardly ever picked up, except by the cleaner when the room was dusted. From this episode, Molly learnt that when something that is precious is lost, even an identical replacement does not eliminate the sense of loss.

Previous loss can also put present losses into perspective, in that emotions may be recognized and a sense of comfort gained from the fact that one does get over even the most horrendous losses and come out the other side. Mrs Wynne is such an example (Ch. 4). She was a lady who, in normal circumstances, made a considerable fuss about even the most minor problems. She hated her family to be late for dinner, and if a cake singed when she cooked it, she was likely to dissolve into tears.

Five days after her son's death, a heavy fall of snow came through the roof and this resulted in Mrs Wynne's bedroom ceiling falling down. In the normal way, this would have been a great disaster, but in relation to the loss of her son it was nothing. In fact, she stood in the bedroom and laughed.

Those who work with bereaved people require warmth, empathy and the skills of effective interaction. Their work will be enhanced if they can use their own losses and their reactions to them to help them in understanding other people's reactions to the most major loss of all, death.

Box 1.1   Requirements for those working with the bereaved

- Warmth
- Empathy
- Skills of effective interaction
- Ability to use one's own losses to help understand other people's reactions to death.

SUMMARY

In this chapter it has been seen that:

- death is a loss and that although many adults have not suffered bereavement, they have all suffered losses of some sort, both in terms of possessions, pets, ambitions and people
- the magnitude of the loss is in relation to the importance of what has been lost and its relative value to the person who has suffered that loss
- society's expectations are sometimes at odds with the reality of the loss from an individual perspective
- every individual can learn from lesser losses and be in a position to use those experiences to help them to understand those who are working through the bereavement of a person whom they loved.

REFERENCE

Simpson M A 1975 Teaching about death and dying. In: Raven R S (ed) The dying patient. Pitman Medical, London

---

FURTHER READING

Alexander H 1993 Bereavement: a shared experience. Lion Publishing, UK
Burnell G 1989 Clinical management of bereavement: a handbook of healthcare professionals. Human Sciences Press

Clark D 1993 The sociology of death. Blackwells

Dickenson D, Johnson M (eds) 1993 Death, dying and bereavement. Sage Publications, London

Dillenburger K 1992 Violent bereavement. Avebury

Duffy W 1991 The bereaved child: A guide for teachers and leaders. The National Society

Faulkner A 1993 Developments in bereavement services. In: Clark D (ed) The future for palliative care. Open University Press, London

Furman E 1981 A child's parent dies: studies in childhood bereavement. Yale University Press, USA

Gersie A 1991 Storymaking in bereavement. Jessica Kingsley Publishers

Gorer G 1965 Death, grief and mourning. Cresset Press, London

Green J, Green M 1992 Dealing with death: practices and procedures. Chapman & Hall, London

Gunzburg J 1993 Unresolved grief. Chapman & Hall, London

Hill L 1994 Caring for dying children and their families. Chapman & Hall, London

Houlbrook R 1989 Death, ritual and bereavement. Routledge, London

Jones M 1988 Secret flowers. The Women's Press

Lewis C S 1966 A grief observed. Faber

Littlewood J 1992 Aspects of grief: bereavement in adult life. Routledge, London

Murgatroyd S, Woolfe R 1982 Coping with crisis. Open University Press, London (Reprinted 1993)

Neuberger J 1987 Caring for dying people of different faiths. Austin Cornish/Lisa Sainsbury

Parkes C M, Weiss R S 1983 Recovery from bereavement. Tavistock Press, London

Penson J 1990 Bereavement: a guide for nurses. Harper & Row, London

Richardson R 1991 Talking about bereavement. Optima

Sanders C 1989 The mourning after: dealing with adult bereavement. John Wiley & Sons

Sherr L 1989 Death, dying and bereavement: an insight for carers. Blackwell Scientific Publications

Sheskin A 1979 Cryonics: a sociology of death and bereavement. John Wiley & Sons

Wallbank S 1991 Facing grief: bereavement and the young adult. Lutterworth Press

---

BOOKS FOR CHILDREN

Buchanon Smith D 1987 A taste of blackberries. Puffin

Hill S 1982 In the springtime of the year

Hoy L 1983 Your friend Rebecca. Bodley Head

Little J 1986 Mamma's going to buy you a mocking bird.

Mellonie B, Ingpen R 1983 Beginnings and endings with lifetimes in between. Dragons World Ltd, Surrey

Sims A 1986 Am I still a sister? Big A & Co., USA

Stickney D 1984 Waterbugs and dragonflies. Mowbray

Varley S 1985 Badger's parting gifts. Picture Lions

2

Facing death

Bereavement is commonly seen as a phenomenon which starts after the death of a loved one. This is certainly true in sudden death where a relative might leave the house in the morning, well and happy with no concerns, and later have a road traffic accident and die. In such a case, the bereaved person's family and friends have no time to get used to the fact that death is going to happen, whereas in terminal illness there is a period where the patient, the family and friends have to face the reality that the time is short and that the loved one is going to die. The bereavement process in this case starts prior to death. How this period of time is handled will have a considerable effect on the pattern of grief displayed by those who are left behind.

THE UNMENTIONABLE SUBJECT

Most people do not think actively of either their own death, or that of those they love. In a healthy society many people do not encounter death at first hand. This is also true for health professionals who often see their first death after they have started preparation for their career. They may see a seriously ill patient deteriorate and die, and feel somehow responsible for what has happened. Added to this is the fact that in our society death is not a subject that is openly talked about. Buckman (1988) suggests that people do not know what to say to someone who is dying or to the person who has been bereaved. A mother who lost her son through a sudden viral infection said that the worst time for her was just after the death when, in the village shop where she had been known for many years, everyone would stop talking when she came in. The bereaved may interpret such behaviour as lack of care, when in reality people do care, but they do not know how to talk about anything as emotive as death.

Illness in ourselves or in someone whom we love confronts us with our own mortality, and if the illness is terminal then there are a number of reactions that can occur as the person attempts to come to terms with a new and possibly frightening situation. The way that each person adapts to the possibility of death of a loved one may have a profound effect on the way that they grieve. Similarly, the way that the patient adapts to their own impending death can colour the memories left for those who will grieve after the death.

DENIAL
A coping mechanism

Denial is a very common and very useful coping strategy for many individuals; for example, if bills arrive before money is available in the bank to pay them it is very common to put the bill in the back of a drawer and forget about it until such time as money becomes available or a reminder arrives. This mechanism is very useful in that it helps the individual to avoid worrying about a particular matter at the time of its arrival. However, what it does not do is to take away the need to accept that one day reality must be faced. Denial of serious illness and the potential consequences poses many problems for both health professionals and the informal carers of the patient, but if it is used as a strong coping mechanism it should be taken away at one's peril because there may be no other coping mechanisms available to the patient.

The costs of denial

The costs of denial are probably greater for those who care for the person in denial than for the person themselves. It is not unusual for a dying patient to ask friends, relatives or health professionals to look at holiday brochures and talk quite excitedly about the holiday they will have when they are better.

Meg: 'I thought we would go on that cruise when I am better'.

Husband: 'OK. Where do you want to go?'

Meg: 'Madeira. We always said we would go'.

Husband: 'Yes. Shall I get some brochures?'

In this example, Meg's husband reinforces her denial but below, a sense of reality is maintained without taking away hope.

Meg: 'I thought we would go on that cruise when I am better'.

Husband: 'It would be lovely if you were well enough'.

Meg: 'Yes. Shall we?'

Husband: 'Let's leave it for now but see how things go'.

If Meg's husband had supported the denial and assured Meg that she would get better, then when Meg realized that she had been fooling herself about the outcome of her illness, she is likely to be very angry with those who colluded with her. These feelings of anger may persist until the death and they can make grieving more difficult for those who are left behind. In addition to this, denial has the effect of halting useful interaction between the dying person and those who are important in their lives.

People who know they are dying generally want to get their 'house in order'. They may talk with those they love, about what they want in terms of funeral, of dealing with their belongings, and of the future that they would hope for those they love. Such planning can be quite a positive experience for the patient, but can be difficult for those who care since it may reinforce a reality that is painful and difficult. It may also engender a range of emotions which relatives and loved ones may feel they are unable to share with the dying person, such as grief, anger, guilt and blame. These emotions are often felt by both the relative *and* the dying patient.

ANGER

Many patients, when faced with a serious diagnosis and an uncertain future, can become very angry—angry because they do not think they have deserved what is happening to them, angry with those who they feel might have been in some way responsible for what is happening to them, and anger at their God for not caring for them in the way that they had thought according to their own religious beliefs. The patient often displays this anger inappropriately. Much of it may be aimed at the health professional; doctors may be accused of late diagnosis or inappropriate treatment, but in fact often do not deserve the anger that is coming to them. Relatives who come to visit the patient can be very upset to find that the person they love is suddenly somebody who is angry and bitter and seeming to lay much of the blame for their present plight on the innocent relative (Faulkner 1992).

FEAR

Many dying patients are very frightened. They do not know what will happen to them, if anything, after death and much of how they adapt to their impending death will depend upon their own spiritual beliefs (Stoter 1991). Such fears will often spark off difficult questions asked both of health professionals and of family and those who love the patient. Many of these questions do not have an answer. It may be, for example, that an individual who has always been very religious is doubting the love of their God because of their current predicament. Such a person may well question the beliefs that they have been brought up with.

- Is there really a God there anyway?
- Is there a heaven, and if there is, what is it like?
- What if this is all there is?

Health professionals will have been taught to refer such questions to the patient's spiritual adviser, but relatives may have great difficulty themselves in trying to deal with questions about 'tomorrow', and 'how will I die?', and 'will I still know that you are all alright?' Very often, bereaved people will remember those conversations and feel guilty because they were unable to answer the questions in an appropriate way.

GUILT

Guilt among bereaved people is considered on p. 41 and may be affected by incidents prior to the death. Patients may also suffer a burden of guilt. Moreover, they do not always feel able to share that guilt with another. Relatives visiting the patient may realize that something is happening but may not understand the nature of the problem. They may need help from health professionals to start a dialogue where there can be an open exchange between the patient who is feeling guilty and the person who loves them. Frequently, terminal disease is seen as a punishment for sins committed and even the most honest and open individuals usually have something in their past which they feel ashamed about, and to which they can attribute their current situation.

UNFINISHED BUSINESS

If a patient is in denial and relatives are colluding with that patient, then there is little chance before the death to allow the patient to deal with any unfinished business. Kubler Ross (1975) talks about stages of adaptation to the fact that an individual is dying. Although these represent a useful paradigm, they do not work for every individual. One of the phases, for example, is anger. Some people are born angry, and they die angry. Others reach a final stage of acceptance where they are prepared to die, or are ready to go.

When a patient does realize that they are going to die, even if they do not accept that this is right for them, they will then start to think about things that they want to do and to say to those they love. Sometimes the relatives are not ready for this, and may block the patient's right to deal with unfinished business. This is difficult for the health professional who sees that both the patient and those who love them have different needs, and the professional may not be sure how to proceed to help both parties.

Some unfinished business is not quite so painful as that illustrated in Box 2.1. When Mrs Melville knew that she was dying, she started giving her treasures to her children. When her elder daughter came to collect her for a holiday 3 months before she died, she realized that her mother was quite ill, and this was

---

Box 2.1   Distressing unfinished business

Joe Smith knew that he was dying: his wife was relatively young, and they had two small children. Joe's major concern was what would happen to his much loved family when he was no longer there to provide for them. One day the staff nurse found Mrs Smith extremely upset, and when she sat her down and asked what the problem was, it appeared that Mr Smith had been asking his wife to consider looking for a new husband after his death. He even suggested a couple of his friends whom he thought would be suitable new partners. Mrs Smith, who still was hoping that some miracle would happen, was distraught to be faced with her husband's reality and also with his desire to look after her, even after he himself would not be there.

---

confirmed by the fact that a picture painted by her grandfather which had always been on her mother's wall, was put into the boot of her car.

'I can't take this Mother', said her daughter and Mrs Melville replied,

'I want to be sure that it's where I mean it to be'.

Accepting family treasures before the death was very painful for Mrs Melville's children at the time, but they knew they were meeting some need in her. In effect, it helped their grieving because they had known that in her last few months, she had done what she most wanted to do.

SAYING GOODBYE

If family members and a patient can talk openly about impending death, there is a chance then that they can say goodbye to each other in a way that suits them all. Many couples live together for years of marriage, jogging along happily together and never feeling the need to tell each other how they really feel. This may suddenly become very important when one of those people is going to die. So often, among bereaved individuals, one hears the comment,

'I didn't even get to say goodbye'.

This most commonly happens when the family are in collusion (Faulkner & Maguire 1994).

PARTNERS, RELATIVES AND FRIENDS

When a patient is dying, then most attention goes to that patient.

The health professionals are offering care and symptom control and those who love the patient are offering their support and care. Until recently, little attention had been given to the needs and reactions of those who love the patient. In terminal illness this is very important. The patient may or may not accept that he is going to die but there is an end to suffering when death occurs. Those who love the patient are still going to be there after the death and have to adapt to that loss.

Isolated siblings

Faulkner et al (1995) in looking at the effects of childhood cancer on the family found that siblings suffer more than the patient in terms of being isolated, feeling unwanted, and feeling almost resentful of the care that their sick brother or sister needed to receive. If death occurs in such a situation, then those siblings are left feeling very guilty that they somehow failed to give the dying person the right sort of love and care when they were able. The feelings that those who love the patient go through prior to the death may have quite a profound effect on the way they are able to adapt to their loss.

NATURE OF RELATIONSHIP

The ease with which an individual adapts to the potential death of somebody whom they love depends very much on the nature of that relationship. In this, many assumptions may be made which in fact are quite incorrect. For example, it is always assumed that married couples love each other and that the impending death of one partner is going to be a life-shattering event for the other. If this assumption is incorrect, then a large responsibility may be put on to the surviving partner to display a grief that they may not feel.

Just as assumptions about the love that exists between people can be incorrect, it is also possible that those who will be most bereft after the death may be missed. There can, for example, often be more love between a woman and her grandchild than there is between that same woman and her daughter. Similarly, there may be illicit relationships, such as a mistress, where love may not be shown in public.

Box 2.2 Death bringing freedom

Mrs Timms had been married for 40 years before her husband was found to have cancer and only a few months to live. In fact Mr Timms had always been extremely mean, both with his wife and with their children. This had caused endless heartache since they were financially comfortable and the meanness was totally unnecessary. Health professionals observing Mrs Timms when visiting her husband were very impressed with the equanimity with which she viewed her husband's impending death. They were unaware that she was not in any way sorry that he was going and that when he died she would feel free for the first time in many years.

EMOTIONAL REACTIONS

The emotional reactions of the patient who is dying may be mirrored in those whom they love. These are:

- fear
- anger
- guilt
- blame.

These reactions may all be present along with the difficult question of

'why should this be happening to somebody that I love?'

As with patients, anger felt by a relative may well be displaced on to health professionals and again, this anger needs to be explored and identified and correctly placed so that the individual may diffuse the anger and recognize its roots (Faulkner 1992).

Causes of guilt

It is not unusual for relatives to feel responsible for the illness and impending death of the person whom they love. In a study of childhood cancer (Faulkner et al 1995), one father felt totally responsible for his child's cancer, because he knew that he had killed innocent people while on active service in the Suez Crisis. It is important that the individual is allowed to talk through these feelings so that they can begin to forgive themselves, and realize that there is not necessarily a link between their guilt and the illness of the person whom they love.

Another very common cause of guilt is the concern that the

dying person has not received enough love—'if only this had happened or that had happened'. The individual does not necessarily feel that if things had been different the patient would not have died, but they may feel that because the patient is dying things should have been different. Many people, for example, save their money for a rainy day. When the person they most love is going to die, it seems too late then to have the fun that they could have had if they had not been quite so worried about potential problems in their lives.

Asking 'why?'

The patient may be asking:
'why me, why do I have to die?'
The relatives are asking that same question but in a slightly different way:
'Why has the person I love got to die? Why am I being deprived of the person who I care so much about?'
The root of the question is often connected with beliefs and spirituality, and may simply indicate a need on the part of the relative to talk through and think of all the things that have and have not happened in their relationship. They will usually be perfectly aware that there simply is not an answer to the question 'why?' but they may well be helped by empathy and acknowledgement of how difficult it is to understand why such a calamity has happened in this family.

COLLUSION

If the patient chooses to be in denial and the family colludes with that, we have seen that there may be repercussions after the death in that there has been no chance to deal with unfinished business or say goodbye. However, collusion sometimes happens when the patient does want to talk about what is happening and the relatives do not. They will make strong arguments that they know the patient best and that the patient could not bear to be told (Faulkner 1992). The health professional will then need to help the relatives to understand the costs of collusion to themselves and then hopefully negotiate to open the whole area up with the patient, who generally has a clear idea of what is happening. The important issue is that collusion usually occurs because of love from the colluder to the patient. They simply cannot face the pain of the patient's understanding that time is short.

It is not always possible to break collusion, and in essence one has to look at the reasons for and against breaking it.

> Rob knew well that his wife was dying, but did not wish her to be told. As a result, his children were not involved either because he feared that they would be unable to keep the secret that their mother was dying (Help the Hospices 1992). When the specialist nurse talked to Rob's wife, she knew perfectly well that she was dying. The conversation went as follows:
>
> Nurse: 'Pam, if you know the way things are and you know Robert also knows, I wonder why you're not talking to each other'.
>
> Pam: 'It's the last gift that I can give him'.
>
> Nurse: 'I'm sorry?'
>
> Pam: 'Well, Rob wants to believe and keep everything as normal as possible. He's turning himself inside out to make sure that our life goes on as far as possible the way that it always has. I can't take that away from him. If I told him that I knew the way things were, then it would all fall apart for him, and I can't do that'.

In the example above, collusion was not broken, and as a result there were post death costs for both Robert and the children. However, both individuals had made an informed choice on how they wanted to behave at the time of Pam's dying. That was their right.

UNFINISHED BUSINESS

Just as the patient has unfinished business to attend to, so do the relatives, and often they find this a difficult subject to broach, especially as the time of death grows near. Typically the subject is broached by the patient or not at all. Yet if a dialogue can occur where the person who will be bereaved knows the wishes of the person who will die, then the subsequent bereavement will be easier to handle. Take for example the following dialogue:

Ron (in bed one evening):	'You alright Amy?'
Amy:	'Yes, I've felt sort of 'lighter' today. You know I won't get better?'
Ron:	'Yes love, I wish it were different'.
Amy:	'It's harder for you—being left behind'.
Ron:	'Oh love'.
Amy:	'Things on your mind?'
Ron:	'The 'after' without you to be my other half. And what I'm going to do with the others. They won't be able to bear it'.

In the dialogue above, Ron was anxious about a future without Amy, but Amy made the dialogue possible where they could both discuss the shape of a future after her death.

Family rifts

Unfortunately, unfinished business where it involves disposal of the dying person's possessions often causes friction within a family, and this is an added cause of silence between the dying person and those who will be left behind. Unfinished business, however, may also include emotional issues within a family. It may be that there is a family member who has been ostracized for some reason in the past, and when another member of that family is dying there is a feeling that the rifts should be repaired. This is not always possible and family members may need to be helped to understand that just because somebody is dying, they are not necessarily going to become any more forgiving than they were in the past.

If the family rift is long-standing, then health professionals have to ask themselves the question as to whether the problem is related to the illness or separate from it, and if it is separate they should not get involved, since it is unlikely that things will change. The ostracized family member, however, may be someone at risk of not being able to grieve within normal parameters, because of the unfinished business between themselves and the person who is dying.

A major difficulty for the health professional may arise if that member of the family arrives to see the patient, and other family members request that they are not allowed in. The responsibility here for deciding whether the patient sees the prodigal member of the family must lie with the patient, if they are able to make a decision. Often these two people, without other family members around, will make their peace. This is an advantage to the patient who dies with one less thing on their conscience, but it is also helpful to the prodigal member of the family in terms of how they are able to handle their own grief.

SAYING GOODBYE

Many people while still in good health promise each other that they will not die alone. This typically happens with young married people who cannot imagine life without each other. What they also cannot imagine is what it is like to be with someone who is dying. It is not uncommon to have the most significant person in the patient's life sitting by the bedside keeping a vigil in the last hours or days that the patient is alive. Many hospices in this country have a family room for just that purpose, and in Holland (Faulkner 1995) the large cancer centre in Rotterdam has a family house so that the people closest to the patient may actually live-in to be with their relative while they are having treatment or, more particularly, when they are likely to die.

So often, however, when someone is keeping a vigil they get tired and eventually need to leave the patient, maybe to have a shower, a meal or a rest. In that period away, the patient may die and this can lead to guilt and remorse that can affect bereavement. It is not possible to take away the ensuing guilt, but it is possible to help that relative to see that they were there right to the end and that their relative would have been aware of their presence. It happens so often that it is also possible to say:
'maybe your relative was waiting for a quiet moment to go'. This is something that is unknown, but does seem to be more than coincidental.

CHILDREN

The whole of Chapter 8 is devoted to the bereaved child. When a close relative is dying, most parents wish to protect their children from the reality until the last possible minute. Children are often simply told that a parent or a much-loved granny or aunty is ill and not told the severity of that illness. The arguments for not telling them are usually due to the belief that the child will be naturally upset, but also that the child will not be able to understand. What the health professional can do to help parents involve their child when someone is dying, is to encourage them to answer the children's questions as they come and to answer exactly what is asked. So, for example, the child might ask first of all:

'Why is mummy always in bed?' but may go on at a later stage to say:

'Will mummy be well again, or is mummy going to die?'

The child will then get the information at the pace at which they can absorb it. They also have a chance to be involved with the dying, to be part of the unfinished business, and to have the opportunity to say goodbye to the person whom they love.

Box 2.3 The child who is involved

The child who adapts best to bereavement is the one who felt involved; like Lucy, who was told that Mummy would not get well and took over the task of finding surprises to take to Mummy in hospital. Later her mother took off her gold locket and put it round the child's neck and said:

'Look after this for me Lucy because I know I can trust you to do so'.

Lucy was five then and is 16 now. She does not even take the locket off when she bathes but she can say:

'This was mummy's and it was the last thing she gave to me'.

ACCEPTING DEATH

It will be seen that both patients and relatives find the period when they have to face death extremely difficult. They may try and deal with this avoidance, by denial, by collusion, and if all these prevail until death, then it can be assumed that grieving will be quite difficult.

If, on the other hand, the reality of impending death is faced, then both patient and relatives and friends have time to accept what is going to happen, to prepare for it, to deal with unfinished business and to say goodbye. This does not mean necessarily that grieving will be easy or that is will be without complication, but it is important to realize that those things that happen before death can have a profound effect on what happens afterwards.

SUMMARY

In this chapter the following have been considered:

- the period before death
- the link between that period, and how it is handled
- the potential effect on the grieving process.

It has been shown that if the dying person, and those whom they love, can accept the impending reality of death, then grieving for the loss of the beloved is more likely to fall within normal parameters.

REFERENCES

Buckman R 1988 I don't know what to say. Papermac, London
Faulkner A 1992 Effective interaction with patients. Churchill Livingstone, Edinburgh
Faulkner A 1995 Cancer centre profile. Journal of Cancer Care 4:2.
Faulkner A, Maguire P 1994 Talking to cancer patients and their relatives. Oxford University Press, Oxford
Faulkner A, Peace G, O'Keeffe C 1995 When a child has cancer. Chapman & Hall, London
Help the Hospices 1991 Child of a dying parent. Video by Screen Productions, London
Kubler Ross E 1975 Death, the final stage of growth. Prentice Hall, London
Stoter D 1991 Spiritual care. In: Penson J, Fisher R (eds) Palliative care for people with cancer. Edward Arnold, Kent

3

After death: the immediate future

Even when the death of a loved one has been expected there is usually a sense of shock when the actual death occurs. This feeling of shock is even more profound if the death was not expected, or if the loved person was in a sense of denial of the impending death. This sense of shock is often accompanied by a sense of disbelief and unreality. The disbelief is less easy to maintain when the bereaved person sees the body, and for this reason, a belief has arisen that all bereaved people should be encouraged to do so.

A SENSE OF UNREALITY

If there is no recognisable body or no body because of the circumstances of the death, then the sense of disbelief may well be maintained over time and actually prevent the individual from being able to grieve. The nature of how the death was presented to the bereaved is usually remembered with crystal clarity. Helen, for example, remembers waking in the night to the telephone ringing and the nurse from the hospice saying,
   'Please come to the hospice. I'm afraid your mother has died'.
Although Helen was expecting her mother to die, she had thought it would not be for several days ahead and had in fact

asked to be with her mother when she died. She was alone in the house and in a great sense of panic as she got into her car and drove to the hospice. She later recalls having no remembrance at all of that car journey. Similarly, some of the relatives of the dead at the Hillsborough disaster in Sheffield were seen driving the wrong way down one-way streets because they were in such a state of shock that they did not know what they were doing.

How to break the news?

Health professionals often feel quite helpless at such times. If someone dies in the night, should they telephone the relatives or should they wait until the morning? Should they telephone a neighbour or ask the local vicar to call round and break the news? In fact, such decisions should be made with the relative before the death if at all possible. Many people will ask to come to the hospital before the death and will sit with their relative. Others feel that there is little they can do and would prefer to stay at home, but to be informed either as soon as the death has occurred or, if the death occurs in the middle of the night, early the next morning.

What does the relative want?

The priority is to find out what the relative really wants as opposed to what they think they should do. Coming to the hospital immediately after a death may seem to be unnecessary, particularly if the bereaved person is on their own and therefore at risk of accident because of their shock. On the other hand, the bereaved person may be desperate to be there with the body, even though the death has already occurred. Some people may gain a sense of comfort from sitting by the dead body for a while.

PRACTICAL MATTERS

Dealing with the practicalities of death can in fact be therapeutic for the bereaved in that it gives them a purpose at a time when they are feeling lost and helpless and sometimes wondering when they are going to wake up. However, many bereaved people find it quite difficult when asked by the hospice or hospital personnel to take away their loved one's belongings, to sign books for them

---

Box 3.1   An apparent lack of feeling

Even when the relative sees the dead body, a sense of unreality may persist. Joanna, coming to see her husband after his expected death, described the experience as follows:
  'It was like being in a dream; John was lying there and he looked like John and yet he didn't. It was like looking into a doll's house, real but not real, and I didn't feel anything'.
  This apparent lack of feeling may in fact be a defence, much as denial is a defence, against being completely overwhelmed by grief without any time to begin the painful adaptation to life without the beloved.

---

and various other administrative tasks. Some people may feel quite detached and totally unable to sort out what they should do next and so they may ask questions about undertakers, funerals, what one needs to do at the point of death. In this respect, funeral directors usually offer good advice and help to the bereaved, so that they can set in train the practicalities of the funeral.

Positive aspects of the practicalities

Practical issues, such as:

- letting other members of the family know what has happened,
- putting an obituary in the paper,
- planning the funeral,
- organizing caterers

may all help the bereaved person to put off the point where they actually allow their grief to surface. At this time too there is generally plenty of support for the bereaved person and their family. Friends, neighbours and relatives rally round and very often give time and attention to those who are grieving. Cards and telephone calls remind the bereaved person and their family

Table 3.1   Services offered by funeral directors

Help with:
  Contacting minister
  Collecting Death Certificate
  Registering death
  Putting death notice in papers
  All aspects of the funeral

---

how much love there was for the dead person, and in many ways this period of time can have positive aspects.

The Chapel of Rest

One practical issue relates to where the dead body is placed prior to the funeral. It is increasingly the practice to take the body directly from the hospice, hospital, or the patient's home to a Chapel of Rest where the undertakers will make the deceased look as attractive as possible. The coffin lid will normally be left off until the day of the funeral. This allows those who have known and loved the dead person to visit the Chapel of Rest and pay their last respects. It also creates a situation where the dead person is distanced from their family, including some who may not see the body (either because they do not wish to or because other family members feel that it would be unwise) and others who may maintain some level of denial.

Viewing the body—an informed choice

This can create problems for children who are protected by their parents and as a result get no chance to see the body of their dead relative. What is important is that all those involved, whether they be children or adults, should be allowed to make an informed choice about whether they wish to see the body after the death. Many would argue that it was much easier in the days when the body was brought home, and put in the coffin on the dining table in the 'best' room so that family members could pop in and sit by the body or look at it at any time they wished up to the point of the funeral.

THE FUNERAL

Whether or not to attend the funeral of a loved person can become an issue. It is traditional that family and friends should attend, partly to say their last goodbyes and partly because of the expectation of society. This expectation does not always include all members of the family. If there have been family feuds, there may be a feeling among some members that other members should not be allowed to attend. As with viewing the body, the important point is that the individual concerned, whether adult or child, should be allowed to make an informed choice about whether or not to attend.

The final goodbye

The funeral serves the purpose of focusing on the reality of death and that this is the final goodbye. The format may vary according to culture and according to spiritual belief, but in all events it marks an ending to life on earth. Bereaved people will often describe the phase from the time of death until after the funeral as a time when they were 'acting on automatic pilot', meaning that they have gone through the ritual of preparing for the funeral without any feelings or emotions breaking through.

Life is made easier for relatives if some indication of the nature of the funeral has been discussed with the patient before they died, particularly in terms of whether they prefer burial or cremation. Some patients who have accepted impending death have already planned their own funerals, while others die without any mention of what arrangements would be their wish. The sense of doing what the loved one wanted may sustain many bereaved people during the planning, preparation, and the actual event of the funeral.

Lack of sensitivity

The funeral itself may be quite a strain for immediate family and friends of the dead person. Painful memories may remain if the event is not handled sensitively, or if there are indications that some mourners do not show due respect. Differing perceptions of what death is all about may surface and raw feelings can be exacerbated.

Christopher carried angry memories away from his young wife's funeral after the Minister had said a prayer:

'Let us pray for the soul of Pat, and remember that we must not be sad because she has been called to God so soon. Let us rather remember that she was so precious to God that he called her to him and gave her grace'.

Positive aspects of ritual

There are positive aspects to the ritual of the funeral, not least the support and love of friends and family. If there are flowers, they are another tangible reminder of love and respect for the dead person.

EMOTIONAL REACTIONS

During the first few days after a death, the bereaved person may experience a number of difficult and worrying emotions.

Searching

One of the most common of these is the often unconscious need to look for the dead person. For example, Anna, whose boyfriend was killed in a car crash, described how for days after the death she found herself at the spot of the accident. She could not recall how she had arrived in the particular street or why she was there, but she was in fact searching and going back to the last place where her boyfriend had been alive. This searching behaviour can be exhibited by multiple visits to the hospice or hospital where the patient died. The bereaved relative will often appear with very small excuses. They may come to ask for an item of clothing that they think is lost, they may bring back articles that they had borrowed during the time of the illness, but what they are really doing is trying to get close to the person who is dead. Because the reaction is almost always experienced at an unconscious level, it can be confusing. The relative does not put on her hat and coat and say,

'I'm going to look for him at the hospital'

but rather she finds herself turning a trivial reason for visiting the hospital into a very important reason for returning, even though at a logical level they are well aware that their partner is dead, and that there is no need for haste.

Believing the dead person is still there

This searching is often linked to a need to believe that the dead person is still there. Often a bereaved person will describe how they were walking down the road after the death and suddenly in front of them they see the beloved. They run to catch up with that person knowing that when they get there the death will all have been a terrible mistake and that their loved one is going to turn round and be there for them. They will describe the sense of desperation and desolation when they reach the person that they have seen, and they turn round and they are not at all the person they were looking for. This is beautifully described by Monserrat in 'The Cruel Sea', in the passage where Lockhart runs down the road, sure that his girlfriend, Julie Hallam, is in front of him. He describes how he feels when the girl turns round and it is not Julie. He knew at a logical level that Julie had been killed in a boating accident, but he was unconsciously searching for her.

Hallucinations

Another common phenomenon after a death is the belief that the dead person is still around. This may manifest itself in hallucinations or may be a feeling that the dead person is not far away. A daughter described how, a few days after the death of her mother, she was going shopping, walked down her front path and found herself waiting with the gate open for her mother to come through before she closed it and went to the village. She knew at a logical level that her mother was dead, but the feeling that she was still there was so strong that she couldn't ignore it. These emotions may be very worrying for those who experience them, and they may be helped to know that they are not uncommon occurrences and are usually only temporary. The concern of many bereaved people is that they are 'going mad'.

'Good copers' and blockage of grief

Although grief is expected from those who have had to face the death of a loved one, society on the whole reinforces non-tearful behaviour. Individuals are seen to be 'good copers' if they appear to be getting on with life as if the death had not occurred. This feeling that the bereaved person should not show emotion is strengthened by the fact that many individuals have no idea what to say to the bereaved (Buckman 1988).

This apparent lack of concern on the part of others may add to the sense of unreality surrounding the first few days after the death,

'If the death had occurred, why don't people talk about it? Maybe it's all a big dream'.

This reluctance on the part of society to talk about death may have an effect of actually blocking the bereaved person's expression of grief, at least in public. They may feel that they are not expected to cry or to show their pain, and so are encouraged to put on a 'public' face of coping. Table 3.2 shows emotional reactions in first few days after a death.

TRIGGERS TO GRIEF

The actual process of grieving is usually triggered by something relatively small. It could be that the death has been accepted, that the relative or partner has worked through the practical matters, the ritual of the funeral, the getting on with life, and will describe themselves as 'having coped very well in a difficult situation' and then something will set them to feeling the pain of grief (Worden 1991).

A bereaved mother who had known that her child was dying felt that she had coped very well with the death and its aftermath, and then she found herself after the funeral tidying up when the many visitors had left. She walked into the sitting room and caught sight of a picture of her dead child. This mother goes on to describe how she sat on the sofa and cried and cried, and felt that she could not stop. She knew that it was the photograph that had triggered her grief reaction, and later explained that it was seeing the picture that reminded her that pictures were the only memories she would have of how her child looked. Other triggers can include suddenly seeing a favourite television programme that a person had always

Table 3.2 Reactions during the first few days after death

Shock:	• sense of unreality
	• feeling 'numb'
	• little show of emotion
Searching:	• largely unconscious
	• often returns to place where dead person was last seen
	• often seeing stranger and believing it to be dead person until face to face
Hallucinations:	• feeling dead person nearby
	• feeling presence
	• hearing voice

watched with the dead relative. Sometimes a snatch of music will take an individual back to being with the dead person, and such events will act as triggers to the expression of grief. This is probably the most painful set of feelings that the bereaved person will have since being told that death had occurred, but they are important in their function of putting an individual in touch with their feelings.

Box 3.2   Triggers to grief

- photographs
- familiar possessions
- favourite places
- TV programmes
- music

SUMMARY

In this chapter, the immediate period after the death has been considered:

- The news that a loved person has died will come as a shock whether or not it is expected, though the shock will be greater if the death is unexpected.
- Many people will describe the phase immediately after the death as one where there was a sense of unreality.
- Some people may find that the practical matters and the ritual associated with death and with burial or cremation may support them through the first few days.
- The first few days may be accompanied by a range of differing emotions that can be quite worrying.
- Society tends to reinforce the feeling that emotions must be hidden and blocked, but eventually for most bereaved people some trigger will set their grief pattern in action.

REFERENCES

Buckman R 1988 I don't know what to say. Papermac, London
Monserrat N 1951 The cruel sea. Penguin, London
Worden 1991 Grief counselling and grief therapy. Routledge, London

The pattern of manageable grief

It was seen in Chapter 3 that after the death of a loved one, many people appear to be in a state of shock. During this period they may describe their feelings as being in a 'blocked stage', and say that they go through the days on 'automatic pilot'. It was also seen that during this period, there may be a number of emotional reactions including searching for the beloved, having hallucinations, or the feeling that the loved one is still around. This period, along with the tasks and rituals that follow a death, may well serve a useful function, in that it gives space and time for the person to adapt to the death.

EMOTIONAL REACTIONS

Fear of mental illness

Just as searching behaviour and hallucinations are an integral part of adaptation, depression may also be a temporary feature. These experiences may lead the person to believe that they are mentally ill, particularly if they have not previously experienced such intense feelings.

Restlessness

Other reactions may add to this belief. For example, some people find that they are extraordinarily restless; they cannot stay in the house, but when they get outside they want to go back. These feelings can be frightening.

> Mrs Wynne's son was in the Air Force in Singapore. He had met and fallen in love with a female colleague while there, and decided to marry her before coming home at the end of his term of service. On the day of his wedding, his family at home in the UK received a telegram which they imagined would say,
>   'Done the deed. Coming home'. Instead it said,
>   'Regret your son died at 7 a.m. this morning. Cause unknown'.

Given that this was an unexpected death, after which the bad news was broken in the starkest way possible, Mrs Wynne was unable to take in what had happened. She could say that she knew her son was dead, but she could not assimilate it and over the next few days her normal routine disintegrated. She did not bother to dress properly, she did not want to cook or clean, and the house suddenly became overwhelmingly claustrophobic. She would ask her husband to take her for a drive to their son's house and then to her sister's house, but once she had been somewhere for a very short time she needed to move on. Her daughter-in-law tried to help her to describe her feelings;

Mrs Wynne: 'I must get off. I must get home'.

Jan: 'But you've only been here about 10 minutes, Mum'.

Mrs Wynne: 'I know, but I just can't stay'.

Jan: 'Why don't you tell me about it'.

Mrs Wynne: 'I think I'm going mad. Last night, I woke up in the middle of the night and he was there at the foot of the bed, I'll swear he was. I got out of bed and of course when I got there, he wasn't there. Then I made a cup of tea; I sat in the kitchen and I looked at the mess—you know how fussy I am—but I can't be bothered any more. I'm not sleeping properly, and I just have to keep moving on'.

Jan: 'Do you know why you keep moving on?'

Mrs Wynne: 'I guess I'm trying to run away from it, and to an extent I do. When I first came here this afternoon to see you, I could almost believe it hadn't happened, and then it's as if it catches up with me again'.

It was very difficult for Mrs Wynne to understand that her deep disturbance was a very natural reaction to what had happened. Her son was buried abroad, so she had no function to plan and no focus to her life during those first, very difficult, days.

A trigger for grief

For many people, the sense of unreality and the accompanying emotional reactions change after a few days as something triggers the pain of grief. For Mrs Wynne it was a letter from the Air Ministry, giving details of the burial and the place of burial of her son. Whereas the telegram had induced a state of shock which left her confused, feeling irrational and wanting to dismiss the message as untrue, the letter put her in touch with the finality of her son's life. She was then able to start crying and to feel the pain.

FEELING THE PAIN

One of the difficulties for those who are bereaved is that there is no clear format of how they should feel or how long they should feel it for. However, they can be reassured that certain reactions are fairly common, and that the time they take to work through those feelings is infinitely variable. For example, the state of shock will happen even when a death is expected, but it is likely to be more profound if the death is sudden. The same applies to the pain level which occurs once the true grief reaction has been triggered.

A natural reaction

Many people will describe crying for days; others will have bouts of crying in between apparently normal behaviour. The temporary depression may persist for a while with individuals feeling unable to sleep, unable to be bothered with daily chores, or often with their own appearance. At this point, many bereaved people go to their general practitioner and ask for sleeping pills. What they may find hard to understand is that they need to feel the pain and that this pain is a natural reaction that has to be worked through after the death of someone whom they loved.

A case of mixed feelings

The onset of these intense feelings which wash over people may be very difficult to cope with. Molly cared for her mother in her last illness; she sat with her at night and stayed with her until she died. After the death she made arrangements for the undertaker to remove the body to a Chapel of Rest and nego-tiated with him to arrange the funeral. Having done that, she went to bed for the first time in several days, had a deep sleep and woke up refreshed.

No feelings of grief

Molly and her sister went for a drive and talked about their mother, but neither of them showed any feelings of grief. There was a lot to do and neither of them really thought about what they were feeling, or indeed of what they should be feeling, given the deep love they had for their mother.

Laughter

Their mother had always loved surprises, and as children they had both enjoyed treasure hunts and egg races at Easter. They were, therefore, not surprised when they looked through her papers to find that the will was not there. Together they searched the flat and in every drawer or cupboard in which they looked, they found a little pot that had money in it. There was one pot full of half-crowns, one full of 50 pence pieces and one full of old sixpenny pieces. Finally, they found the will in a black blanket box that their mother had had ever since she had been married. Both women sat on the floor and laughed. It felt exactly as if their mother was there.

Tears

Suddenly, sitting on the floor by the blanket box which smelled of the mothballs that their mother had always used, Molly started crying. It was totally uncontrollable and she felt as wretched as she had ever felt. She also felt extremely confused— how could she have been laughing minutes before, such a short time after her mother's death, and now feel as desolate as she did? She saw her own behaviour, from the time of death to the time of finding the will, as almost bizarre and was quite convinced that she was going mad.

Molly explained the story to her general practitioner and asked for sleeping pills.

Molly: 'I just need something to help me sleep for a few nights. The whole thing's been so bizarre—I'll never forgive myself for laughing so soon after she died'.

GP: 'Well, you've had quite a heavy time during the last week or two. How much sleep have you had?'

Molly: 'Well, that makes it worse. OK, I've been up with her a lot, but once the undertaker had taken her away and I'd tidied up a bit, I just went to bed and crashed out and slept like a baby. How could I do that?'

GP: 'I suspect that your body needed you to do that'.

Molly: 'And then believing that mother had set up a treasure hunt for us!'

GP: 'Well?'

Molly: 'I suppose it took us back years. Yes, I'm sure that's what it was, but we laughed. It's silly really. I guess while we were going round the flat and finding all the ways that she'd been squirrelling her money away, we were reminded. I guess during that time we weren't really believing that she was dead'.

GP: 'Well, I think that's how it is and maybe that was a bit of a safety valve for you while it was happening'.

Molly: 'But now?'

GP: 'Now you've got some really hard work to do because you've got to get in touch with that pain, and you've got to work through it. It won't be easy and I hope you'll understand when I tell you that sleeping tablets won't help you'.

Molly: 'But I need something'.

GP: 'You need to do your grieving'.

ANGER, GUILT AND BLAME

Of the many emotions experienced after a death, anger, guilt and blame are probably the most common, and can be very confusing.

Anger

Inappropriately focused anger

Often, after the news of a death, the bereaved person becomes very angry. This reaction may be general and clearly linked to the perceived unfairness of the death, or it may be inappropriately focused. This may result in misunderstandings in the family, and the bereaved person may be perceived as unkind.

Within a few hours of hearing that her son was dead, Mrs Wynne turned on her husband and said,

'Why wasn't it you, you've had your life. His was just beginning'.

Mr Wynne was very upset by this comment, since he was also feeling the blow of his son's death. What he did not understand was that his wife's anger did not really belong with him and that she certainly did not mean that she wanted him dead. Her anger actually lay with the God that she had always believed in, who appeared to have let her down by stealing her son.

Justifiable anger

Occasionally after a death there is justifiable anger as, for example, when someone has been murdered or has committed suicide. The bereaved relative or loved one may well feel very angry with the murderer or with the dead person for taking their own life. Working through the anger, whatever its cause, is a part of the grieving process. However, the angry person may need help both to focus and to diffuse the strong feelings (Faulkner 1992).

Guilt

Similarly with guilt, death commonly brings on the 'if only' syndrome in those who loved the dead person, as they consider all the things that they should have done for their loved one if only they had realized that time was so short. This guilt is often unfounded and unnecessary, but it can act as a mechanism whereby the bereaved person makes sense of what has happened.

Blame

Along with guilt, or in place of it, there are often feelings that the death would not have occurred if someone else's action had been different. It is very common, for example, to believe that if an illness had been diagnosed earlier, the patient would have recovered instead of dying. The focus of blame is often inappropriate and short-lived, but it is an integral part of the emotional reactions to death.

Loneliness, sadness and physical pain

Anger, guilt and blame are some of the emotions that are part of the pain of loss. They may come and go over the first few days after a death, and some may linger on. They will be linked with other emotional reactions, which may include loneliness, incredible sadness and feelings that are akin to physical pain.

PLATEAU

One of the problems for many people is that when their pain is triggered, they may feel overwhelmed and begin to believe that they will never ever feel normal again. They are frightened that their distress will consume them. For most bereaved people this period of very intense feeling lasts for only a few days before the grief plateaus. This means that the person will get on with their life, but will continue to have heavy feelings of sadness with bouts of intense feelings washing over them. Some may feel so depressed at this time that they really feel that life is not worth living. These feelings are within normal parameters in the early days after the death of a loved one, but the majority of bereaved people do begin to feel better, albeit slowly, and over a period of some weeks.

SLOPE

Figure 4.1 shows this progression from the initial shock of hearing of a death, through to some improvement that shows that the individual will start to recover. However, recovery can be the cause of another set of problems for the bereaved. If the dead person was much loved, they may feel that intense grief should be sustained over a prolonged period of time.

Just as most people can identify the point at which their pain was triggered after the initial shock of death, so they can identify the turning point where the pain began to feel a little less.

Mrs Wynne: 'I still feel really sad and sometimes I still wonder if it's true. If anyone mentions his name I cry'.

Visitor: 'I can see just how upset you still are, but I wonder is there anything that's happened in the last week or so that's allowed you to know that things might get a little better?'

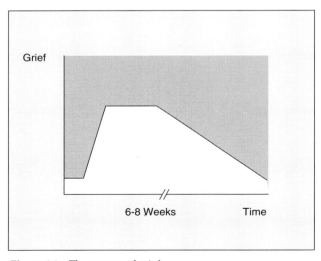

Figure 4.1   The pattern of grief

Mrs Wynne:	'Well, I suppose I'm sleeping better, but that's because I make myself work hard all day. I find that if I do things, then I can keep going and I've been doing some spring cleaning. It sounds silly but I just have to keep on the go'.
Visitor:	'Are there any other changes?'
Mrs Wynne:	'Well, his box of things came home—I suppose it must be 3 weeks ago—and a couple of days ago I managed to open the box and start sorting his things'.
Visitor:	'And how was that?'
Mrs Wynne:	'It was terrible, but I managed, and I guess if I'm honest I couldn't have managed it before. That box has just stood as it was delivered, so yes, I guess I'm moving just a little bit, but God, it hurts'.

In the above sequence, Mrs Wynne could identify two areas in which she knew that she was moving on in her grief;

• She had been able to start sorting her son's things which she found very painful.
• She was beginning to sleep more normally than she had in the first few weeks after her son's death.

However, once a person begins to feel a little better, a sense of guilt may creep in. They may wonder how they could possibly begin to feel anywhere near normal so soon, and they may feel that they should remain on the plateau of grief as a mark of respect for the dead person. The first few indications that a slope is beginning to occur may be almost unconscious, and the first good night's sleep after a death may well be seen as a bonus. Providing that the bereaved person is able to talk through these feelings, they will generally continue moving, albeit slowly, down the slope towards feeling able to pick up the threads of life again (see Table 4.1).

SETBACKS

Once a person has started on their slow recovery, they may be relieved by the better feelings that they are having. Finding that

Table 4.1 The grieving process

After death	Feelings
Shock	Feeling of disbelief
	Searching
	Hallucinations/feeling dead person present
Trigger to pain	Waves of intense feeling
	Anger, guilt, blame
	Temporary depression
Plateau	Pain continues but at more manageable level
	Can distract for increasing length of time
Slope	Can identify more positive feelings
Setbacks	Grief reactivated by anniversaries or triggers, but not at original level

they can laugh when they thought they would never laugh again can increase the feeling of well-being, even though it brings with it some guilt feelings. Sleeping properly and being able to distract from the pain of grief are also signs of recovery, but the bereaved individual must expect some setbacks.

Anniversaries

Anniversaries and special occasions are often triggers to setbacks. The first birthday after the death of her son was a very sad day for Mrs Wynne. She woke remembering that it was her son's birthday and found that she was crying. Her immediate reaction was that all the good work that she had done in adapting to her loss was undone, and that she was back at square one. In fact, she was still on her slope and the pain on the birthday did not take the grief back to its original level. Her next bad day was on her own wedding anniversary and she felt totally unable to have the usual family celebration on that occasion.

There is a theory that the first set of anniversaries are the hardest for the grieving person and that once those are through after the first year, then things should be considerably easier. This does not mean that there will not be occasional setbacks, so bereaved people need to understand that these feelings may go on for a very long time, even though the death has been accepted, and the grieving has been worked through.

Revival of grief

Box 4.1   Trigger for a revival of grief

Alice's husband had died of a heart attack, aged 45. Very soon after that, a family friend's wife died under tragic circumstances. Their son had died of leukaemia and she had not been able to deal with the aftermath and so had committed suicide. Alice often went to the friend's house taking cakes or a pie to help Doug along. Doug, the family friend, reciprocated by mending the washing machine and doing the small repairs that Alice's husband used to do.

Eventually, Alice and Doug fell in love. They both felt they had worked through their grief and they were ready to get married. Two years after they were married, Doug's daughter was visiting her father and student tenants had just left the home which Alice had shared with her first husband. She asked Doug's daughter to come with her to look at the house, to see what work needed to be done.

When they arrived at the house, Doug's daughter walked round the garden to see if it needed any immediate attention. After a while, she thought she would go into the house and make a cup of tea for her step-mother. As she arrived on the doorstep quietly, she was appalled to find Alice standing by the sink with tears rolling down her face.
    'Whatever is the matter?' she asked. Alice replied,
    'It's his (her first husband's) birthday, but please don't think because you've seen me like this that I don't love your father'.

Being in the house that she had shared with her husband and in which they had brought up their four children, Alice was remembering their life together as she walked round. When she went to the kitchen and saw the calendar, she remembered that it was her husband's birthday, and the combination of factors triggered a revival of her grief.

Over time, the potential for such triggering becomes less in most bereaved people, but it is a reminder that although somebody is dead and no longer in their lives they are not forgotten, nor yet are the feelings that they had for that person forgotten. What happens is that the feelings are put to one side so that the individual is open to new relationships, as Alice had been open to the new relationship with Doug (Box 4.1).

TIME

When a person is feeling the pain of grief and working through the associated feelings, they often worry about how long the pain will last. This is a very difficult question, in that the time that it takes to be open to new relationships is very variable and depends on a number of factors. These include:

1. How close the relationship was, and how committed the two people were to each other.
2. The individual's lifestyle and how big a part the dead person played in that life.
3. How significant the dead person was compared with other relationships.

Away from home

Mrs Wynne's son had been abroad for 2 years prior to his death and had not been home during that time. Her contact with her son was mainly by airmail letters and occasional postcards. At anniversaries and on special occasions, parcels of interesting mementos would arrive from Singapore. In the early days after his death, the postman would be a trigger, and could induce tears but as time went on and Mrs Wynne learned not to expect anything from her son any more, she adapted to the postman not bringing airmail letters.

It could be argued that Mrs Wynne's day to day life was little affected by her son's death. Her feelings of sadness and despair were for a son who was adult and had virtually left home. This did not affect the level of her grief, but it did affect her adaptation to life without him. Her setbacks came at times when he would have been uppermost in her mind, such as on anniversaries and special occasions. Her level of grief was reactivated by the appearance of the girl whom her son would have married, for her presence highlighted the absence of her son.

Part of day to day life

If the dead person has been a significant factor in day to day life, like a spouse or a child, then it could be argued that the adaptation to life without the loved person will take considerably longer. Again this is not in terms of the level of the grief, but more to do with adapting to day to day living and the potential for triggers.

SUPPORT

An important element in the way that an individual copes with their grief is that of the support they receive, and the perceived reactions of those that are within the family and social circle of the bereaved. Mr Wynne coped very differently with his grief compared with his wife. The telegram about his son's death appeared on a Saturday, and Mr Wynne went back to work on Monday morning. His wife saw this as a lack of caring, but he perceived it as a method of coping. He argued that life had to go on and that a living had to be earned. His pragmatic approach to this difficult situation led his wife to believe:

1. that he had not cared for his son,
2. that he did not care for her.

As a result she looked for her support to her daughter-in-law who had two small children, and it was her daughter-in-law who helped her to see that although she and her husband coped in very different ways, this did not affect the way that they both had felt about their much loved son. What was important to Mrs Wynne was that she was able to talk through her feelings and get them into some sort of perspective.

SUMMARY

In this chapter the pattern of manageable grief has been described:

- In the early days after a death, the emotional reactions often lead to an individual believing that they are going mad as they find themselves searching for the loved one, hallucinating that the loved one is present and suffering from temporary depression.
- These emotional reactions will become part of feeling the pain of the death of the loved one and will include anger, guilt, blame, sadness and loneliness.
- After a few days of intense waves of feeling, the grief will plateau for a while and gradually turn into a downward slope as the individual begins to adapt to the death.
- There will be setbacks, particularly at anniversaries or times when the loved person would have been very much in the foreground of the bereaved person's life.
- For those who cope with their grief within manageable limits, the slope is generally reached around 6–8 weeks after the death, though there is considerable variation in this time.

REFERENCE

Faulkner A 1992 Effective interaction with patients. Churchill Livingstone, Edinburgh

5

Assessing a bereaved person

Most people who are bereaved cope well with their grief. They may be deeply unhappy for a considerable period of time, but with the support of family, friends and others, they will adjust to their loss. However, a small proportion of bereaved people break down after bereavement and are referred for psychiatric help (Murray Parkes 1972). Between those that cope without outside help and those that need psychiatric intervention in order to cope, there is a group of people who could be helped by some outside agency, other than family or friends.

PEOPLE AT RISK

With current resources it would be quite impossible to visit every bereaved individual, but prior to the death, factors may be identified which allow those 'at risk' of being unable to cope to be followed up after bereavement (Ch. 6). These risk factors should be taken into account. However, they are at best a rough guide as to those who will or will not cope with their grief.

Limited resources

One could argue that if a person was not coping well, there are outside agencies such as Cruse to which they could refer themselves. However, it has to be accepted that bereavement intervention in our society is far from adequate (Clark 1993). Because of limited resources, intervention with bereaved individuals should be targeted at those most likely to have problems. This means that the first visit to a bereaved person should be one in which the individual is assessed to discover if their grief is within those limits that can be handled by the person themselves with support from family and friends. Table 5.1 shows main areas to cover in order to make a useful assessment.

TIMING

It was seen in Chapter 3 that immediately after a death the person is in shock, and likely to be experiencing difficult and

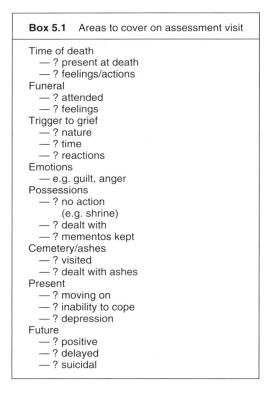

Box 5.1 Areas to cover on assessment visit

Time of death
— ? present at death
— ? feelings/actions
Funeral
— ? attended
— ? feelings
Trigger to grief
— ? nature
— ? time
— ? reactions
Emotions
— e.g. guilt, anger
Possessions
— ? no action
    (e.g. shrine)
— ? dealt with
— ? mementos kept
Cemetery/ashes
— ? visited
— ? dealt with ashes
Present
— ? moving on
— ? inability to cope
— ? depression
Future
— ? positive
— ? delayed
— ? suicidal

painful emotions. At that point, what they seem to need most is comfort from those who love them and from those who have cared for the patient. Often a bereaved person, when describing the period immediately after death, will say how helpful it was to have the local general practitioner (GP) come in and ask how she was. Similarly, in order to gain this comfort the bereaved person may well go back to see the staff who cared for the loved one. This may be in the form of an excuse such as bringing in the funeral flowers, or something similar that makes the visit to the ward acceptable to everybody. Thus we can distinguish between this need for comfort and the searching behaviour described in Chapter 3, where people find themselves returning to the last place that they saw their beloved for a trivial reason which suddenly becomes very important, or for no logical reason that they can explain either to themselves or to anyone else.

A willingness to talk

The assessment visit should concentrate on whether the bereaved individual has in fact started on the slope of normal grief (p. 42), no matter how small that slope may be. This is generally happening by 6–8 weeks after the death, and by then, typically, there is a willingness to talk about the bereavement and resultant feelings. Earlier is often a little too upsetting for many people who may describe their current state as being so confused that they do not know where they are going. Also, by 6–8 weeks after the death, if the reaction is one of clinical depression, the symptoms are generally clearly discernible.

NEGOTIATION

It cannot be assumed that everyone who is bereaved will welcome a visit from someone who wishes to help them, be that person a member of the health care team who cared for the patient, a volunteer from the institution in which the patient was cared for, a member of the clergy or a member of staff from the community if the patient was nursed at home. The assessment visit is more likely to be welcomed if the bereaved person knows that the visit is to take place and has agreed to the time and the place. It is also helpful if the length of the visit is negotiated so that it does not compete with other demands on the person's day.

The casual approach

Many health professionals feel that if one negotiates the time, the place and how long the interview will last, somehow this will distance the bereaved person from the visitor by being too 'cut and dried'. It is further argued that a bereaved individual has so much to be coping with, that they should be given the impression that the bereavement visitor has all the time in the world for that one person. In fact such an approach diminishes the importance of the individual by assuming that they are free to spend a considerable amount of time, at no notice, talking to the visitor. Consider the following interaction:

Nurse Jones: 'Hello Mrs Meredith. You'll remember me, I looked after your husband when he was dying. Just thought I'd pop round and see how you're getting on'.

Mrs Meredith: 'Well . . .'

Nurse Jones: 'Can I come in? I must say you're looking better'.

Mrs Meredith: 'Well, yes'.

Nurse Jones: 'Shall I come through here?'

Mrs Meredith (looking at her watch):
                 'All right dearie. How are they all at the hospital?'

Nurse Jones later reported that Mrs Meredith was distracted and seemingly not very well adjusted to her loss. In fact Mrs Meredith was reasonably well-adjusted. She was still feeling sad and missing her husband considerably, but her rather negative behaviour when she saw Nurse Jones was due to entirely different reasons. One was that she had children to collect from school soon after Nurse Jones appeared and was very flustered as to what she could say without seeming rude, and secondly, part of her coping mechanism was to bury herself in day to day matters so that she actually had no desire to talk through the way that things had been. If Nurse Jones had negotiated, she could have managed a different time slot and given Mrs Meredith the chance to say if she thought whether it would be helpful to talk about her husband's death and its aftermath.

A more positive way

Negotiation can be seen in a much more positive light than in the previous illustration. It allows the bereaved individual to be part of the decision making as to whether or not they wish to talk. Similarly, by being given a time for the visit, they have a clear idea of how long a potentially painful interview will last. They are also much more likely to agree a time which will fit in with other aspects of their day, without feeling that they have to make other arrangements for domestic chores or issues.

The open-ended approach is threatening

The notion of 'all the time in the world' may sound caring and may give the impression that the patient matters tremendously to the person coming to visit. However, 'all the time in the world' may also be seen as threatening, in that talking about loss, particularly a recent death, can be traumatic. Such an open-ended approach might make some people too frightened to actually agree to being visited.

A further positive message is given if, as part of the first visit, negotiation relates to the future. For example, a nurse might ring a bereaved relative as follows:

Nurse Porritt:	'Hello Mrs Meredith. This is Nurse Porritt from the hospice. It's 7 weeks now since your husband died, and what we like to do here is follow up the partners and see how they are coping. Would you be prepared for me to come round?'
Mrs Meredith:	'Well, well I suppose so'.
Nurse Porritt:	'You don't sound too keen'.
Mrs Meredith:	'Well, I'm not sure about raking it all over. How long would you want to come for?'
Nurse Porritt:	'Probably just half an hour to start with, just to check how things are with you, and to see if you need any further help. After that visit you may not need to see us again, but if you do then one of us will come back and review after a few weeks'.

The above can be interpreted in negative terms—only half an hour and the possibility of only one visit—but in fact there is a positive message here; firstly, that the nurse is aware that the relative may only feel able to talk for a limited time without getting too upset, but more importantly, that the feelings of grief will change, allowing adaptation so that in the future Mrs Meredith will not need the professional support that is available. It will be seen in Chapter 10 that such negotiation protects both the nurse from building a dependency relationship, and the relative from becoming too dependent on an inappropriate person.

LANGUAGE

In an assessment of a bereaved individual, the person them-selves may find difficulty in talking about the death and its aftermath. This difficulty will be compounded if the bereavement visit does not use language that is explicit. So often it is thought to be kind to use words such as 'loss', or phrases such as 'passed over' when what we really mean is dead. Nurse Porritt, in the telephone call to Mrs Meredith clearly stated,

'It is 7 weeks since your husband died'.

This made a clear distinction between an assessment visit and a friendly visit from a relative or near neighbour to see how the bereaved person is. Death in our society is still one of the taboo

---

Box 5.2 The tasks of grieving

Worden (1991) sets out the tasks for a bereaved individual. These are important for those who work with the bereaved, because they state quite clearly where the responsibility for grieving lies, namely, with the bereaved individuals themselves. Further, the tasks give the parameters for stages in accepting the death of a loved one. The tasks are as follows:

- accepting that death has occurred
- feeling the pain
- accepting life without the beloved
- being open to new relationships.

These tasks can help the bereavement visitor in identifying where the individual is at in terms of those tasks and to assess the level of recovery from whatever feelings of grief they are experiencing.

words and as long as professionals, friends and family use euphemisms rather than the word 'dead', the relative is not being helped to face up to a reality of death.

THE INDIVIDUAL'S PERCEPTIONS

The purpose of an assessment interview is to identify whether the individual:

1. is coping well enough with support from loved ones that they will work through their grief without further aid from outside agencies,
2. needs some further help in order to cope,
3. is so disorganized by their grief that they require specialist help.

In order to distinguish between these three possibilities, it is necessary to ask the individual to talk about their perceptions of the death and its aftermath up to the point of the bereavement visit. The assessment needs to be carried out in a sensitive manner, but nevertheless in a way that will clearly identify how the person is coping.

DEATH

Even if the bereavement visitor was present at the death, it is important to ask the bereaved person how they now perceive the events around the death. This encourages them to talk about how they felt at the time they knew that their loved one had died and how they felt immediately afterwards. They may describe the sense of unreality and some of the emotions described in Chapter 3, and this is often followed by the statement,
'I felt as if I was going mad'.
That this statement is made in the past tense will help to identify if the person has truly accepted the death and come away from the sense that this is all unreal and perhaps a very nasty dream.

One can argue that discussion of the death may be far too painful for the individual to talk about, but people usually describe feeling much better after they have talked through their feelings, and put them into some sort of perspective to a non-judgmental visitor who will be able to reassure them that they were not going mad and that what they describe are common phenomena. It is true that such a description may be distressing, especially if it is the first time that the individual has had a chance to describe how they felt. Society does not generally encourage such disclosures as illustrated below.

Nurse Porritt: 'Mrs Meredith, can you tell me how you felt when you knew that your husband was dead?'

Mrs Meredith: 'Well dear, I didn't really feel anything, that was what was so strange, you know. I knew he was going to die and I was worried about letting myself down when he did by crying and being upset, but I wasn't. It was quite amazing, I just . . there was just nothing. OK, I knew he was dead. It was after that was so awful'.

Nurse Porritt: 'What was so awful?'

Mrs Meredith: 'Oh, I couldn't keep away from the hospice afterwards. I kept finding myself at the gate. I stopped myself going in but I used to keep going there and I couldn't understand it. Sometimes I even believed that he was still in there. I really thought that I was going mad'.

Nurse Porritt: 'But you feel differently now?'

Mrs Meredith: 'Oh yes, yes, I know he's dead. Yes, I know I was a little mad but it's OK now. I guess I'm not unusual, am I?'

Nurse Porritt: 'Well, you're very special and unique, but what you are describing does happen to a lot of people'.

Mrs Meredith: 'But you know everybody told me how well I coped. I guess I was able to hide it pretty well'.

Nurse Porritt: 'And how did that leave you feeling?'

Mrs Meredith: 'Well, I didn't feel a lot then, I just kept saying to myself, "He's dead, you've got to accept it and he isn't coming back".'

THE FUNERAL

Helping an individual talk about the funeral gives them a chance to express concerns, but it also gives a clear indication of their attitude to the death and its aftermath by their willingness to plan and attend the funeral, or their inability to go there because it was all too distressing. If an individual has difficulty in accepting a death, then the funeral may have the function of underlining the reality that death has occurred. There may be problems of adaptation if there is no body and if no ritual takes place such as a funeral or memorial service.

In fact the period between death and the funeral is often so full for the bereaved person that it allows them, perhaps unconsciously, to shelve their true reactions. They may have quite a lot of organizing to do in terms of getting family members together, arranging for cars, the flowers, the type of coffin—a number of things that will totally absorb them, and many bereaved individuals will describe this in fairly positive terms, for example in the dialogue below.

Mrs Meredith: 'In a way I was glad that there wasn't anybody else to organize the funeral because it kept me occupied. When I was talking to the vicar about the service, he asked me what David's favourite hymns were, and do you know, I could talk about that without crying. It was as if I was still on some sort of 'automatic pilot', sorting out the food and what was suitable, and then the flowers. The undertaker was such a kind man and yes, I coped. It was quite amazing how I coped'.

Nurse Porritt: 'And the funeral itself?'

Mrs Meredith: 'Well, yes, I woke up that morning and I didn't really want to go, but I had a public face on I suppose, so yes, I did it. I even arranged all the sandwiches and everything before we went, and I didn't cry. I was surprised at that. It was almost as if the sense of unreality was still with me. You know there was the music and the sunlight coming through the church windows. It was strange but I went, but I don't think it struck me then that he'd really gone'.

For Mrs Meredith the funeral was a ritual that helped to keep her going without getting her in touch with her true feelings about the death of her husband. For many individuals the funeral underlines the death and causes considerable open grief at the ceremony.

If the individual has attended the funeral, it is very important to identify the reasons for this and to judge the effect on the person's likelihood of grieving within normal limits. It is possible to be so upset by the death that going to the funeral is an absolutely insurmountable hurdle, and this needs to be differentiated from the relative who did not go to the funeral because:

a) they are not a churchgoer and
b) they felt that they said their goodbyes before the death.

AFTER THE FUNERAL

It can be seen that the funeral represents a time when families get together and support each other over the death of their loved one, but after the funeral life goes back to where it was before. Relatives return home, the telephone calls get less, the cards stop arriving, and the bereaved person is very likely to suddenly realise just how empty life will be without the person who has died.

In asking a bereaved person to describe that period, it is often possible to identify the trigger to the expression of grief starting in terms of Worden's second task, feeling the pain.

Nurse Porritt:	'And after the funeral, Mrs Meredith, you said you coped very well throughout. You didn't cry in church, you did all the arranging, but what about afterwards?'
Mrs Meredith:	'Well, it was just so quiet afterwards, they'd all gone. I went back into the house and I just didn't know what to do'.
Nurse Porritt:	'What did you do?'
Mrs Meredith:	'Well, I thought I'd tidy up and that was a mistake'.
Nurse Porritt:	'A mistake?'
Mrs Meredith:	'A mistake because I went into the spare room and there was David's photograph. I cried. I sat on the bed and I cried. It seemed that I cried for hours. It just suddenly struck me that all I'd ever have in future was a picture and memories'.

It can be seen that what happened to Mrs Meredith and what happens to many bereaved people, is that they contain their grief until a point when something, usually something very small, triggers the grief reaction. With Mrs Meredith it was a photograph of her dead husband. Her response to the photograph was spontaneous and painful, since it faced her with the realization that her husband was dead in a way that his death and the funeral had not.

In helping the person to describe this triggering and subsequent grief reaction, the bereavement visitor will gain a clear picture of the depth of the reaction, the length of time that it lasted and also what, if anything, has changed since that time. In allowing the individual to describe their feelings, sometimes how they cried for days, or how they still are crying at night, one of the important areas to identify is when the grief started to plateau (p. 41) and if the slope has started. It is very useful to ask the question,

'Is there any way that you can see that tells you that things are even a tiny bit better than they were? '

Sometimes this brings out a sense of guilt, for example:

Nurse Porritt: 'You say that when you saw that photograph you sat on the bed in the spare room and you cried. What happened after that?'

Mrs Meredith: 'Well, I just seemed to be crying most of the time. I got on with what I had to do, but sometimes it was too much trouble getting out of bed in the mornings and some days I didn't even bother to dress. I just felt this awful sadness all the time. I didn't go in the spare room any more. I didn't take the photograph away, I just shut the door and over the next few days—oh well—it was just so awful'.

Nurse Porritt: 'And is there any way now that you know it's not quite as bad as that?'

Mrs Meredith: 'But it should be as bad as that, shouldn't it? It's only 7 weeks and I loved him. We were married 38 years'.

Nurse Porritt: 'It sounds as if you feel a bit guilty. Is it that things are a bit easier?'

Mrs Meredith: 'Well, yes. It was silly. The other day I heard a song on the radio and it was one that was a bit special for him and me. I found myself humming it, almost light-heartedly, and I felt so guilty. How can I be singing when he's only been dead for 7 weeks?'

In the above exchange, it can be seen that Mrs Meredith was beginning to find things marginally easier, but along with that came a sense of guilt. It is important to recognize how hard it is for a bereaved person to face the fact that while they still feel the pain, they may be now moving on to accepting life without the beloved. This is epitomized in a snatch of one of Barbra Streisand's songs,

'The hardest part is knowing I'll survive'.

That song was describing a broken love affair, which is in itself a bereavement even if the ex-lover has not died.

POSSESSIONS

A clear indicator of whether the individual has accepted the death and the fact that life will go on is their attitude to the loved one's possessions. If everything is cleared out immediately after the death, this is as worrying as if nothing is changed. The typical reaction of someone who does not wish to accept the loss of a loved one is that their room is kept exactly as it was when they were alive. It is rumoured, for example, that Queen Victoria, after the death of Prince Albert, had his room kept exactly as it had been during his life, and she continued to have his suits pressed and cleaned, and shaving water put into his rooms in the mornings. This is rather an extreme reaction, but many people who cannot accept that death has occurred may well turn the beloved's room into a shrine and refuse to have things moved. The important factor here is timing.

Being too hasty

Rob's wife was rushed into hospital. She had had a history of cancer and had finally had to be admitted to hospital with brain metastases. She died soon afterwards. The following morning, friends of the family moved in to help the bereaved husband while he went to register the death and make other arrangements. They cleared the living room of all signs of Pam. They folded up the wheelchair and put it away and they collected the books she was reading. Her slippers and dressing gown were all folded up and put away.

When Rob returned, having registered the death, he was very angry and got all the things out again, set them where they were and when he was asked why he had done that, he said,

'It's too soon, I can't let her go yet.'

Spontaneously after the funeral, he himself tidied those things away.

Mementos

It is useful to help the individual to describe not only what they did with the things, if anything, but also how they felt when doing it. This again locates feelings and can be quite helpful. It may be that some things were more difficult to deal with than others. Hopefully, mementos will be kept and sometimes things will be saved to hand on to children or others, but the important thing is that the possessions have been dealt with, or plans made to deal with them in the very near future.

THE CEMETERY

It is helpful to find out if the bereaved person has been able to visit the cemetery if the body was buried, or if there is a special place that they go to if the body was cremated. If the body was cremated, it is important to know what, if anything, has happened to the ashes. Again, it is important to note the extremes. The individual who visits the cemetery every day, sometimes talking to the person as if they were there, is not likely to be coping very well with their loss. On the other hand, the person who goes along occasionally with flowers and gets some sense of peace or reassurance from visiting the cemetery is more likely to be coping within normal limits.

There are of course exceptions. Some people simply do not feel comfortable in a cemetery. To them, once their loved one is dead they are more comforted by looking at photographs, recalling memories and reliving happy times, rather than visiting what they see as an impersonal place with lots of old and mouldering gravestones.

CREMATION AND THE ASHES

If the dead person has been cremated, there is a range of possibilities as to how to deal with the ashes, but what is crucial is that the individual has faced the fact that these are the remains of their loved one and has found something acceptable to do with them. Many people have the ashes scattered in a designated garden of rest. They may pay for a plaque to be put in that place with the details of their loved one on it, or they may have a rose tree planted.

Scattering the ashes

Other people may not wish to do that. Mrs Woodruffe had worried before her death about the fact that her children were located around the country and were liable to move. She made it clear that she did not want her ashes left in some garden of rest where no-one would ever remember to go. Because her family were distressed, they did not ask her what her wishes were. So when the funeral was over, the family discussed the matter. It was suggested that the ashes should be scattered along a river bank where Mrs Woodruffe had often walked. It was a place where her children remembered lovely times. The experience was painful for the son who agreed to scatter the ashes, but somehow he felt very close to his mother while he was doing it, and the rest of the family continued to see that river bank as a special place with happy memories of their mother.

If, in response to the question,
'Have you done anything with the ashes?' the person says,
'Well, not really. They are still in the garage', or
'They are still in the boot of my car',
this again is a warning that the individual may not be handling their grief within normal parameters.

THE PRESENT

It may be quite painful to take a person through from the point of death to talking about what they have done with the possessions and whether they are able to go to the cemetery. Even so, many bereaved people thank the visitor for giving them the chance to talk in an open way, since they may not have had any other opportunity to do so.

Clinical depression

An essential part of the assessment is to identify how the individual is coping at present. If they are able to describe the events in terms that show there is some movement towards adaptation to the death, then they probably can talk of the present in reasonably positive terms. However, it must be remembered that one of the reactions to death is clinical depression and in asking someone to describe how things are at present, it is possible to identify whether or not the individual is clinically depressed.

Nurse Atkins: 'Sounds as if you've had quite a lot of difficulty accepting the death of your wife. How are things for you now?'

Mr Blake: 'Not too good really. I still haven't been to the cemetery. I still find myself doing silly things, like in the morning I'm half way up the stairs with two cups of tea, and I suddenly realize I only need one. I still cry a lot'.

Nurse Atkins: 'What else is difficult for you?'

Mr Blake: 'Well, I don't sleep. I go to sleep when I go to bed, but when I wake up in the morning, often my heart is thumping, and I can't get her out of my mind. When I wake up, sometimes I find I've got my hand out to touch her like I used to, and she isn't there'.

Nurse Atkins: 'And what about other aspects of your life?'

Mr Blake: 'I don't bother much. It all seems too much effort. Silly really, isn't it?'

Nurse Atkins: 'Sounds as if you sometimes think it isn't worth going on'.

Mr Blake: 'Well it isn't. If I wasn't such a coward I'd do myself in. After all, I'd be with her then wouldn't I?'

It can be seen in the above sequence that Mr Blake was not accepting the death of his wife. He was clinically depressed and had suicidal thoughts. This puts him into the range of people who are not going to cope with their grief without specialist input.

Coping

In contrast is Mrs Meredith.

Nurse Porritt: 'Sounds as if, although it's been difficult for you, you are managing reasonably well'.

Mrs Meredith: 'Well, I suppose I'm a bit of a coper. It hurts, I can't tell you just how much it still hurts to know that he's not there, but I am managing and sometimes I catch myself being—well—almost happy. I think of something that we did together when he was alive and I get that warm feeling that I always used to have when he was around. OK, I feel guilty, but at least it means I know that there is something better ahead, and I can go to the cemetery OK. It doesn't always feel as if he's there, but it's a tranquil place and I enjoy putting his favourite flowers there. It's a time when the rest of the world isn't there so I can actually think about him in a positive way'.

Nurse Porritt: 'And now?'

Mrs Meredith: 'Well, I'm not sure if I should feel like that, but I know I am coming out the other end. It'll be tough, it feels tough, but I know I'm looking forward'.

THE FUTURE

A clear guide as to how an individual is coping with the death of a loved one is the way they view the future. It will be seen that Mr Blake did not really see a future and had he been brave enough he would have committed suicide. Mrs Meredith, on the other hand, can see a future and is beginning to look forward. These cases represent the two extremes and there are a whole range of emotions in between. By asking about the future one can get some indication of the level at which the individual is adapting. For example, Marina, an unmarried elderly daughter who had lived with her mother for many years, was looking quite positively to the future 2 months after her mother's death. For the first time in her life she was going to try and find a training programme that would allow her to earn her own living, even though her mother had left funds so that she would be comfortably off.

New beginnings

Sometimes, in talking about the future, other facets of the relationship between the dead person and the bereaved individual will emerge. For example, Mr Horncastle, when asked how he saw the future, talked about a relatively new relationship. The bereavement visitor thought this was rather odd so soon after the death of his wife whom he had cared for with much compassion. In investigating these feelings, it transpired that in fact Mr Horncastle's wife had been ill for a number of years and that he had reached a point where he felt trapped in the relationship. Much as he had loved his wife, he felt that her death marked the possibility of a new beginning for him. He was loathe to talk about this because of the belief in society that everybody who dies was much loved and that they should be properly mourned.

SUMMARY

In assessing a bereaved individual, the aim should be to identify whether that person has accepted the death, begun to feel the pain and begun to move towards accepting that there is life without the dead individual (Worden 1991).

- Asking the bereaved person to describe how they felt at the death, how they handled the funeral and how they felt in the aftermath, will begin to give a picture of how that person is coping.
- This will be helped by finding out how they have dealt with the bereaved person's possessions, whether they have been able to visit the cemetery or a special place, or deal with the ashes, how they view the present and whether they see a future.
- It will then be possible to identify whether the person is on a

slope to show that their grieving is within normal parameters, whether they are beginning to cope but need more help, or whether they need expert help to deal with the feelings surrounding the death.

• The format of the funeral may vary according to culture and according to spiritual belief, but in all events it marks a goodbye to life on earth. Bereaved people will often describe the phase from the time of death until after the funeral as a time when they were acting on automatic pilot.

• Life is made easier for them if some indication of the nature of the funeral has been discussed with the patient before they died. Some patients indeed have already planned their own funeral, while others die without any mention as to what will happen afterwards. The sense of doing what the relative wanted may sustain many bereaved people during the planning, preparation and the actual event of the funeral, and in working towards adaptation to life without the loved one.

REFERENCES

Clark D (ed) 1993 Issues in palliative care. Open University Press, London
Murray Parkes C 1972 Bereavement studies of grief in adult life. Penguin Books, Harmondsworth, Middlesex
Worden 1991 Grief counselling and grief therapy. Routledge, London

6

Inability to cope with grief

Although most people who lose a loved one through death cope reasonably well with support from their family and friends, a small proportion have problems in adapting to the loss. Parkes (1986) differentiates between those who cannot cope with grief because of the consequence of a number of circumstances which all contribute to the outcome, and those where one factor may appear to be the chief determinant of the method of grieving.

For the first type, he gives the example of a young woman with a previous history of psychiatric illness whose husband died suddenly and unexpectedly. The factors affecting her grieving were her youth, her predisposition to mental illness, and a lack of opportunity to prepare herself for bereavement. His example of the second type is Queen Victoria , and the major circumstance affecting her grieving is said to be her strong dependent attachment to Prince Albert.

RISK FACTORS

It is argued here that there are four main areas where those working with the bereaved should take note (Table 6.1). These are:

1. the nature of the relationship
2. the nature of the death
3. the nature of the involvement in the death
4. the past history of the bereaved individual.

Table 6.1 Risk factors

Nature of relationship	Over dependent Stormy Skewed

Nature of death	Violent
	Suicide
	No body
	Sudden
	Senseless — murder
	           — accident
	           — child

Nature of involvement	Has not — visited before death
	        — said 'Goodbye'
	        — seen body
	        — attended funeral

Past history	Other losses — divorce
	           — death
	           — burglary
	           — mutilating surgery
	           — job loss
	Psychiatric history

NATURE OF RELATIONSHIP

The nature of the relationship, whether stable or not, is bound to make a difference to the response of the bereaved person when death occurs. For example, the woman who has been in a strained and difficult relationship for a number of years may actually feel relief at the death of her partner, whereas a young couple deeply in love and consumed with that love may have more problems if one of them is going to die. Those individuals most at risk of being unable to cope with their grief fall into three main categories.

Overdependence

It was suggested earlier in the chapter that Queen Victoria was very dependent on Prince Albert throughout their married life.

She was said to feel upset if he were away, even for a short time, and so she can be cited as someone whose grief was affected by this strong dependence on another person. The major problem here is that if a couple are over-dependent on each other, this tends to have the effect of pushing out the possibility of other close friends and associates. It therefore follows that when one of this partnership dies, the other one not only feels the loss deeply, but also has very few people to turn to for comfort and to help them in working through their grief.

Stormy relationship

Conversely, those in a stormy relationship also appear to be at risk should one of them die. Friends and family may watch them fighting and feuding and constantly bickering with each other, and wonder why one of them does not leave, and yet if one of them dies the other seems to become a pale shadow of their former self.

Mr and Mrs Mount had such a relationship. He was a man who had many relationships outside his marriage and was regularly down at the pub with his mates. He would come home with these friends, sometimes late at night, and occasionally would get his wife out of bed to make coffee for them. His wife would come downstairs muttering and grumbling while she made the coffee. When Mrs Mount had a sudden serious illness and died, her husband was totally disoriented by his grief and was himself dead within a year of his wife's death.

Skewed relationship

A skewed relationship is one in which the feelings and emotions toward the other person are more appropriate elsewhere. For example, if a marriage is going stale and a new baby is born into the family, the baby often grows into a child that brings back some of the excitement of the former relationship with the partner. It might be that the child is bright and bouncy and makes its mother laugh, makes her feel comforted, and makes her feel loved. If that child should then die, the loss is compounded by the strength of the feelings that the child and the parent had towards each other.

A similar situation can occur, but is far less likely to be

identified, when the relationship is extra-marital. It may be that one partner is perfectly happy with the other, but appears to need the excitement of an outside affair. If the object of the attentions outside the marriage then dies, the person left grieving is in a doubly difficult situation; firstly, the strong feelings that they had which more readily belong with their partner cannot be admitted and secondly, the grief must not be shown. This person is at particular risk of not being able to cope with their grief within normal limits.

NATURE OF DEATH

If someone gets a serious life-threatening illness, has some understanding of what that illness might mean and time to adapt to the fact that they might not recover, then those who love that person, providing they have adequate information, will stand a better chance of coping with their grief within normal limits than those who are faced with sudden, unexpected death. This does not mean that people in those circumstances will all grieve within normal limits, for other elements may affect their reaction to the death. It is, however, a fact that the nature of the death can have an effect on the way a person grieves. Those working with the bereaved will normally have some understanding of how the death occurred and it is important to check out how they reacted to the type of death. Much will depend on whether the bereaved person can make sense of what has happened. For example, if a young lad who has repeatedly driven a motor cycle dangerously finally has an accident and dies, his grieving mother may have considerable insight into the fact that what has happened was bound to happen one day, and so the death will make sense to her even though she is grieving and sad that it has happened.

Suicide

Murder or suicide, however, seldom makes sense to those left behind, and the fact that there is no apparent reason for what has happened can make grieving considerably harder. For example, John Avery was 16, one of the brightest boys in his year at school. He was expected to go on to University and had a brilliant future. He had a new girlfriend and lived within a very stable family.

One day John was found in his parents' car with the tube from the vacuum cleaner taking exhaust fumes into the car. Because he left no note and because up to the time of his death he had apparently been perfectly happy, there was absolutely no explanation for his death. This caused his parents enormous problems in terms of wondering whether it was something to do with them that had caused his death, or whether indeed they had missed something about his behaviour in recent weeks. Their ability to grieve within normal parameters was very much affected by the senselessness of the death of someone with such a bright future.

Murder

The grieving is equally hard with the murder of seemingly innocent people. This is particularly true when a child is murdered. Sometimes the murder is accompanied by violation of the body through rape and abuse and those left behind to grieve are often affected by visions of what has happened to their loved one immediately before the death.

Where there is no body

A particular problem arises for those who are grieving when there is no body. It may be that the person has drowned and the body has not been recovered, or in war time situations the only knowledge of death has been a telegram that says, 'Missing, believed dead'. It is very easy for those that love the dead person to fantasize that the death is not a reality and that some day they will return.

NATURE OF INVOLVEMENT

Box 6.1   Dealing adequately with grief

The people who are likely to deal most adequately with their grief are the people who have:
• known that their loved one is going to die,
• spoken freely with them before the death,
• said their goodbyes,
• subsequently attended the funeral for the final goodbye.

The ideal in Box 6.1 is not always met. If, for example, there is no body then it is difficult to feel that goodbyes have been said, and indeed the grieving person may feel that they do not want to say goodbye on the chance that the dead person will return one day.

Collusion and denial

If collusion and denial have been maintained until the death, this can well cause problems for those who loved that person because they have not had their chance to say goodbye and find out what their loved one wanted for the future. In such cases it may well be difficult for the bereaved person to grieve within normal limits immediately after the death because there will be so many regrets and 'if onlys' getting in the way.

Attending the funeral

Attendance at the funeral may become an issue, particularly for children who are often barred from attending in order to save them from distress. Those children who have not been allowed to attend the funeral will probably have more difficulty in coping with their grief than those children who have been allowed to make an informed choice as to whether or not they wish to attend.

Some individuals are so disorientated by the death of someone that they loved dearly that they feel unable to go to the funeral. This can cause problems later on if they regret the chance to have said goodbye to the person whom they loved. This may be compounded if the loved one died abroad and the bereaved person did not make the journey for the funeral. There may have been very cogent reasons as to why the bereaved person could not attend, but in retrospect it is very likely that they will forget this and remember only that they had let down the person they loved by not going.

PAST HISTORY

At a first bereavement assessment, there are signs that the person who is bereaved is not coping well with their grief, then problems to do with the nature of the relationship, the nature of the death and their reaction to it, and the nature of their involvement around the time of the death will give quite good indications of whether this person is going to cope within their own natural resources.

Other losses

By asking about past history, other relevant features may arise that are blocking the individual's ability to grieve. It is very rare for those who are grieving to be affected in their grief by just one factor. Indeed, Murray Parkes (1986), in citing Queen Victoria's dependence on her husband, could have looked for other factors which made the grieving more difficult. It may be, for example, that there had been other losses in the past that had not been adequately dealt with.

The loss may not necessarily be death. Janey Walton was married at 18 to a childhood sweetheart. They were very happy in the early days and when they had been married for 18 months, Janey became pregnant. Her baby was stillborn and soon after that the couple split up. By then the relationship was extremely acrimonious. Later, Janey met and married an older man who seemed to fill her every need. She looked back on her first marriage as a youthful aberration and had never really grieved for the stillborn child.

Janey and her new husband had no children in the 10 years of their marriage before he suffered a violent heart attack and died suddenly. Janey was devastated by her grief and only after exploring her past history did the nurse who was visiting her after the death realize that what Janey was grieving was an amalgam of her early love, her stillborn child and the fact that she had not had children with her new husband. These factors all exacerbated her reactions to the death of her husband.

Emotional baggage

Every individual carries emotional 'baggage' that is not always visible to those around them. Most individuals have suffered a number of losses and have not always been able to grieve in the way that they would wish. This 'baggage' can have a profound effect on any current loss.

IDENTIFYING PROBLEMS IN GRIEVING

If a first bereavement assessment visit is made 6–8 weeks after the death (Ch. 5), it should be possible to identify factors that give an indication that the individual is not coping well with the death of their loved one. It may be that there are prolonged post-death emotions present or, at the other end of the continuum, there may be no post-death emotions. A third observation may be that there are swings in emotions leaving the individual feeling very confused.

PROLONGED POST-DEATH EMOTION

It was seen in Chapter 3 that immediately after a death those that are bereaved report being shocked to the extent that they have a sense of unreality. This may be accompanied by hallucinations, searching behaviour and after a while quite strong emotions such as anger, guilt and blame, as they try to make sense of the death of a loved one. Most of these emotions fade after a period of time. For instance, it is unusual to have hallucinations for more than a few days after a death, and the same may be applied to searching behaviour. The anger, guilt and blame that come with feeling the pain of death usually also fade with time.

Unable to say goodbye

However, the above is not true for all bereaved people. Hallucinations and searching behaviour might continue for a considerable period of time.

> Mr and Mrs Hollis had been married for 50 years before John Hollis died. A year after the death, Mrs Hollis was regularly seeing a grief therapist because she could not rid herself of the belief that John was still a part of her life. She knew that he was dead, but could not accept that he had left her, and so she talked about him in the first person and talked to him. Her therapist was working on a programme where Mrs Hollis was learning to say goodbye to John. A nurse asked her one day how successful the grief therapy was.
>
> Nurse: 'Yes, but what about you?'
>
> Mrs Hollis: 'Well, when I'm with the therapist I say goodbye to John because I know I've got to give him up one day'.

Nurse:	'And how's it leaving you feeling?'
Mrs Hollis:	'Well dear, you know what it's like—you know I go there and he's pleased with me and I do what he asks me to, but when I get on the bus—well, John and I do laugh'.

It can be seen that Mrs Hollis had not adapted to the loss of her husband. However, she was not unhappy. In terms of Worden's (1992) tasks she certainly had not accepted the death, even though she was able to say, 'I know my husband is dead'.

Chronic grief

For other people, the searching stops as does the belief that the dead person is still present. They move on to Worden's second task of feeling the pain, which may include the emotions of anger, guilt and blame, and their emotions may plateau after a few days. However, some people do not start a slope towards adaptation to life without the other person. When asked how they feel in comparison to immediately after the death, they will say that their feelings have not changed. They may still be crying themselves to sleep at night and they will describe the intensity of their pain as being unchanging. Such descriptions suggest a situation which is generally labelled chronic grief (Fig. 6.1).

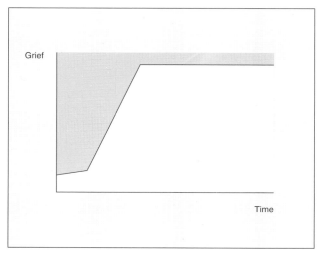

Figure 6.1 Chronic grief

If such a person continues to describe no change in their level of grief and no change in their emotions, then they may need to be referred for more specialist help where they can be guided and helped to move on to a slope of adaptation. In a study of childhood cancer (Faulkner et al 1995), a father was still grieving his child's cancer at a level that had been sustained over a number of years. He was still angry that the child had been diagnosed with cancer. His primary emotion was of extreme guilt for he felt that his child's disease was a punishment for the fact that he had killed people in active service during the Suez Crisis. He still had suicidal thoughts and was advised to seek psychiatric help.

ABSENT POST-DEATH EMOTIONS

Some individuals exhibit no post-death emotions. They do not talk about the immediate post-death time as unreal, they do not describe feeling the pain and they do not describe emotions such as anger, guilt or blame. They may or may not admit that the person is dead. This absence of post-death emotions can be conscious or unconscious.

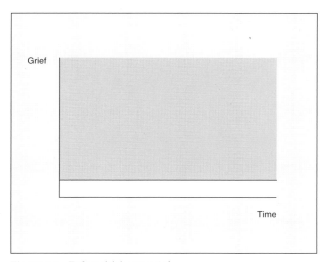

Figure 6.2 Delayed/absent grief

Conscious

When there is a conscious absence of post-death emotions, this may be labelled 'delayed grief' (Fig. 6.2). At assessment, the bereaved person will say that yes, they know their loved person is dead and then give very cogent reasons as to why they may not give in to their emotions. Typical is the young parent who has lost their partner and has small children. Vicky Sims is an example of this reaction.

Vicky: 'Do come in, but I have to tell you the children will be home from school in half an hour or so, so I haven't got long'.

Visitor: 'Well, as I said to you on the 'phone, we like to come round 6–8 weeks after a death just to see how you're coping'.

Vicky: 'I'm coping. I have to'.

Visitor: 'But I wonder if we can talk about how it was for you when your husband died?'

Vicky: 'He died, and yes—of course, there's all sorts of things, but I'm a mother. My children have lost their father and the last thing they want is a weedy wet. I guess you must understand that and at the moment I just don't have time to give in to those feelings. I've had to put the lid on, I don't have any choice'.

Vicky was deliberately delaying her grief, feeling that her children needed her to fill the role of both parents and to be cheerful and available for them. She was able to put the lid on her feelings for the sake of her family in the immediate period after the death.

Unconscious

Some individuals do not display post-death emotions and this is labelled absent grief (Fig. 6.2). Sometimes grief is absent simply because the individual concerned does not believe that death has occurred. This is particularly true when people are killed in active service during war where there is no body and it is possible for the bereaved person to believe that some day the missing person will turn up. They may convince themselves that the idea that their loved one is dead is in fact incorrect.

Blocked grief

Grief may also be absent because it is being blocked by some very strong emotion. For example, Chris (Help the Hospices 1992), at no time talked about the death of his mother for the first year. He appeared to be behaving quite normally and was doing extraordinarily well at school. However, on assessment a year after his mother's death, it appeared that he was very angry with his father because of the nature of his mother's death.

Chris had not been told that his mother was dying, he had not been allowed to be involved in helping her in her last days, he had not been allowed to see the body and he had been sent to school on the day of the funeral. His anger was so monumental that it had totally blocked his ability to grieve, and on further exploration it appeared that much of his anger also belonged with his mother who had colluded with his father to give the belief that life was going on as normal, and that one day she would be better.

At risk

Whether absent post-death emotions are conscious or unconscious, they do leave the bereaved person at considerable risk, for one day something may happen that will trigger their grief, not necessarily in the most appropriate way or place. The resultant emotions are labelled 'exploding grief' (Fig. 6.3).

The trigger to exploding grief can be relatively small. It may be a subsequent loss or it may be something almost intangible such as a smell or a snatch of music. The longer the period between the death and the trigger to exploding grief, the more serious the reaction is likely to be.

Mrs Downs' husband died at a time when her children were very young. She consciously decided that she could not give in to her emotions and firmly put the lid on her feelings about her husband. The longer she repressed her feelings, the more it became unreasonable for her, in her own estimation, to give in to her feelings of loss.

One day a stranger knocked on her door with her dead cat in his arms. Subsequently he had to go to a neighbour's house saying that he was very sorry that he had killed what was, in effect, a scruffy old cat but he could not deal with the owner who was having hysterics next door. What he could not know was

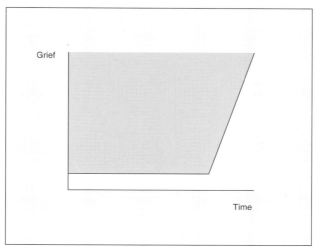

Figure 6.3 Exploding grief

that the cat had triggered the emotions that had properly belonged to the death of her husband.

SWINGS IN EMOTION

The graph for reactions to grief within acceptable parameters (p. 42) gives the impression that after those few days of unreality, a trigger suddenly shoots the feelings of pain to a high level before plateauing over a period of time, and then beginning to move downwards in a slope towards adaptation. In fact in the first few days of grieving, most individuals will describe enormous waves of pain in between small periods of stability.

Many people, however, continue with these waves of pain interspersed with feelings that are often described as quite normal over a period of time, so they do not plateau as is more generally noticed, but continue to have waves of pain over a longer period of time. This is called 'oscillating grief' (Fig. 6.4), and is thought to be conscious in that when the person feels the pain, they become afraid to give it full expression and deliberately suppress it. Eventually the grief explodes and may cause clinical depression and usually requires referral on for more specialist help.

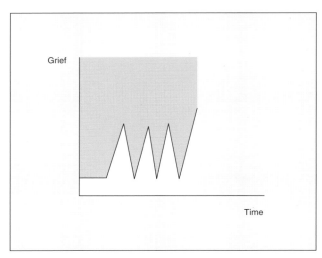

Figure 6.4   Oscillating grief

THE ROLE OF ASSESSMENT

It was seen in Chapter 5 that there are a number of areas that it is necessary to cover in order to make a decision about how the bereaved person is coping (Table 6.1). By exploring each of the areas, it will be possible to pick up those people who are not coping well with their grief. For example, the person who has not accepted that death has occurred, may not have been to the cemetery or dealt with the ashes of their loved one.

Similarly, when asked what they have done with the loved one's things, the bereaved person may describe having left them all exactly as they were. The room may be left as a shrine for a considerable period of time and the bereaved person may still be performing small duties that are no longer appropriate now that the loved person is dead.

Some bereaved people may continue to talk about the dead person as if they were still alive. For example, Lucy fell in love with James. She became worried about their relationship when, after several months, although talking about his parents a lot, he never offered to take her home. Further, as their relationship appeared to be getting closer she felt that he was deliberately drawing away from becoming too involved.

In fact, James' mother had died a few months before he met Lucy. He could not accept that she had gone, and blamed himself considerably for not seeing enough of her before the death. He continued to talk about her in the first person, and it transpired that his reluctance to become too involved with Lucy stemmed from his belief that if he loved somebody, they might die. These feelings and his inability to put his mother into the past tense were in fact early signs of an inability to cope within normal parameters.

By asking the bereaved individual about the future, again it will be possible to pick up those people who are not grieving within normal limits. If, for example, the bereaved person cannot see a future without the loved one then further assessment should be made of their mental state to screen for clinical depression and suicidal thoughts.

DEPRESSION

In those individuals who have difficulty in adapting to the death of a loved one, the temporary depression, commonly experienced, may continue and develop into clinical depression, which will need active treatment.

Table 6.2 Identifying depression in bereavement

After death	Symptoms
Consumed with grief	Low mood Cannot distract Sleep pattern disturbed Poor concentration Cannot get in touch with positive feelings
Negative feelings about self	May feel responsible for death Strong sense of guilt
Restlessness	Constantly on move—trying to escape reality
Withdrawal	Refuses to see others Does not want to talk May sleep excessively
Anger	Anger (may be misdirected) out of proportion in relation to death
Wishes to join dead person	Suicidal thoughts

The symptoms which may indicate clinical depression in a bereaved person are shown in Table 6.2. If four or more symptoms are present, the individual should be referred on for specialist help (Faulkner & Maguire 1994).

The level of pain experienced by an individual can also be assessed 6–8 weeks after the death. The person, for example, who finds talking at all too painful or just impossible may be having problems and the person who shows no emotion may also be at risk. By careful assessment and further in depth enquiry, it should be possible at 6–8 weeks after a death to identify those people who are going to need considerable help in order to adapt to their loss.

SUMMARY

In this chapter, the risk factors of those who may be unable to cope with their grief without experienced help have been identified. These include:

- the nature of the relationship,
- the nature of the death,
- the nature of the involvement in the time around the death,
- the past history of the bereaved individual.

There are clear indications when grief is outside manageable limits. These indications include:

- evidence of prolonged post-death emotions,
- absence of post-death emotions,
- swings in emotions over a longer period of time.

Finally it has been seen that the role of assessment is crucial in identifying those individuals who will need considerable help and expertise beyond that of the average nurse or volunteer who works with bereaved people.

REFERENCES

Faulkner A, Maguire P 1994 Talking to cancer patients and their relatives. Oxford University Press, Oxford
Faulkner A, Peace G, O'Keeffe C 1995 When a child has cancer. Chapman & Hall, London

Help the Hospices 1992 Child of a dying parent (video). Screen Productions, London
Murray Parkes C 1986 Bereavement: studies of grief in adult life, 2nd ed. Pelican, London
Worden 1992 Grief therapy and grief counselling. Tavistock Publications Ltd, London

Grief within the family

When help is offered to a bereaved family, the focus is normally on the individual seen to be most significant to the dead person. This may be a spouse or a child, or indeed a parent. It is relatively easy to make assumptions about which person in the family is most likely to be distressed, and to ignore subsequently other family members whose need for help with their grief might be as great, if not greater, than that of the person who is identified as being most in need.

Perhaps the most common assumption of all is that the person who has died was much loved by the most significant person in their life. This is not always the case and considerable problems can arise at the time of death and in the weeks that follow as individuals within a family attempt to come to terms with a wide range of emotions.

FAMILY PROBLEMS

Most families have problems of one sort or another. It may be that there are several children in the family, one who is seen to be more loved than another by the siblings, or indeed there may be a prodigal child who is not approved of by the whole family. Parents do not always agree with each other, and there are often conflicts between mother and father over how the children are brought up and about the way that the family works together, if indeed they do. Taking the wider family context, there may be conflicts between different branches of the family. It may be, for example, that one member of a family has quarrelled with another, and that there has been a long-standing feud about some quite trivial matter. Conversely, many people have very little to do with members of their family once they have grown up and left home. They may meet on rare occasions, feel fond of each other, but are not a major factor in each other's lives.

Responsibility for conflict

The impending death of a significant member of a family and the death itself can bring many problems to the surface. Health professionals may have to deal with some of these problems as they encounter quarrels between visitors to the dying person and it is often imperative to identify a family spokesperson so that the difficulties within the family do not escape into the health care scene and upset other patients. In such situations, the responsibility for what is happening in the family must be accepted by those members.

Mr Rutter, a businessman, was a patient in the local Hospice. His wife visited every afternoon or evening, and his secretary visited at lunch times with letters to sign from the office. All was well until Mrs Rutter visited unexpectedly one lunch time.

Mrs Rutter: 'Who let that b. . . . in to see my husband?'

Sister: 'Miss Hope is a regular visitor'.

Mrs Rutter: 'It is his mistress—he promised it was all over—she mustn't be allowed in again'.

Sister (gently): 'Mrs Rutter, this has to be a matter between your husband and yourself'.

In the above sequence, Sister refused to take responsibility for the dynamics between Mr Rutter, his wife and his secretary but she did talk to Mr Rutter.

Sister: 'Your wife was very upset today'.

Mr Rutter: 'I guess you think I am some kind of monster'.

Sister: 'No, but I do think you have some serious decisions to make'.

Mr Rutter: 'I know. I'm making both of them unhappy and I'm no good to either of them'.

Mr Rutter went on to talk of his feelings about his short term future, but accepted responsibility for keeping his wife and secretary apart.

Old quarrels

Death may also be seen to bring the family closer together. Old quarrels may disappear, and the family give a concerted effort to making the last days of their dying relative as happy as possible. Unfortunately, this does not always occur. The impending death of the family member may widen rifts and cause bigger problems. What is important for the health professional, is to identify those problems that are directly linked with the impending death and its aftermath from those that have been long-standing. It is too easy to work to the Kubler Ross (1972) paradigm and to expect the patient to die in acceptance with close family members all around. Although a useful model, family dynamics are usually more complex than this.

FAMILY EMOTIONS

Each family member will grieve in their own way and be affected by the unique dynamics between themselves and the dead person. These will include:

- the closeness of the relationship
- the events prior to the death
- the factors around the death itself including the level of involvement of the family member.

There are, however, a number of emotions that may be common to the whole family.

GUILT

Guilt is a very strong emotion and very common at times of death. It may be felt by individuals for things done or undone (Ch. 4) for which they feel personally responsible, but also by families, particularly if the person who has died was in some way a burden to the whole family.

> Mr Avery lived on his own and survived his 90th birthday. He had a home help, he had friends in the village who made sure that he was helped with his shopping each week, and in general there were few problems. He had two children, both of whom lived some distance away, and a grandson who lived within the vicinity. When Mr Avery was dying, he did grumble a little that his children had not offered to have him into their home. There were good reasons for this. He had throughout his life been a very difficult man and although his sons were attentive, phoned him regularly and visited on a very regular basis, they both were in families where their partners and themselves were working, there were small children around and they did not feel that it would be in anyone's interest to take Mr Avery into their home.

> Mr Avery died as he would have wanted to. He moved one evening from his chair where he had been watching television. As he was preparing for bed, which was in the same room on the ground floor, he suddenly had a pain in his chest and when he sat down again he simply crumpled into the chair and died.

> The next morning, the cleaning lady found Mr Avery dead in his room and called the doctor. The sons were called and both felt extraordinarily guilty that their father had died alone without any help from them, either during his old age or at the time of death. The general practitioner talked to the elder son, Alan:

> GP: 'Well Alan, your Dad did it. Looked after himself till the day he died'.

> Alan: 'But he shouldn't have had to'.

> GP: 'But he was all right. I wish all my patients were as well surrounded by loving people as your father'.

> Alan: 'I'll never forgive myself and I know that John feels the same'.

In the above situation, there really was not a problem; a difficult old man had managed with good support to look after himself until the day that he died. His family had been attentive while not taking him into their homes, but the resultant grief was made worse by the guilt that somehow there should have been something else that they could have done.

A typical reaction from the health professional is to tell the family member not to feel guilty. This in fact is not useful. What has to happen when someone feels a high level of guilt is for them to have the opportunity to talk through why they behaved as they did and whether, with hindsight, they can forgive themselves for behaving in such a way.

This sense of guilt often comes about when grief has been triggered. This can be called the 'if only' syndrome—

'if only we'd invited dad to stay with us',

'if only I hadn't been so impatient with him that day before he died',

'if only I'd gone to see her then'.

BLAME

Guilt often leads to blame, since blame is one way to assuage personal guilt. For example, Anna Murray's son was at university when she discovered that she was dying from metastases following her breast cancer. Chris went home regularly to see his mother, but he was very busy studying and was quite happy to be led by his father, who told him that it would please his mother more if he achieved good grades than if he were to visit more often than was reasonable. The week that his mother died, Chris rang his father and talked about coming over to see how his mother was. His father advised him not to do this, but to wait until after the important exam that was taking place at the end of that week. The day after the exam, Chris phoned his father again only to find that his mother had died that night.

At first, Chris felt very guilty that he had not visited his mother, but later transferred that guilt into blame of his father for refusing to face the truth with him. Because Chris was not seen to be the most significant person in his mother's life, no-one picked up his confusion and worries about his mother's death. He continued at university to talk about her in the first person as if she were still alive, and his girlfriend was unaware of the recent death. Within the family, Chris and his father had little to do with each other and neither of them talked about their feelings.

ACCEPTING REALITY

When someone is dying it is common to remember all the good things about them, and sometimes to build a myth that this loved person who is dying was little short of perfect. A problem arises in many families when, in the aftermath of death, this image of perfection is shown to be flawed.

Unexpected disclosures

Ellen's elderly father died and in order to save her mother from the heartache of going through his things, she offered to tidy them out one day a few weeks after the death. Ellen was surprised when she found a bunch of letters in the back drawer of her father's filing cabinet. She took them out, undid the ribbon and found that not only had her father had a love affair, but that it had lasted for many years. The most recent letter was lying in the back of the drawer outside the original bundle, and was dated only a few weeks before his death.

Ellen's first reaction was to take the letters to her mother. She was horrified that the father whom she had always understood to be loving and caring and totally single minded about her mother had in fact had this deep affair. Ellen did not need bereavement counselling, but she did need the opportunity to talk about her feelings and about the costs of either telling her mother and causing her distress, or indeed of holding the secret to herself and perhaps coming to terms with it through talking in a counselling situation.

In fact this sort of situation within a family, causing immense heartache and secrecy, is not always as desperate as would first appear. Ellen's mother was a sensible woman and intelligent. She had known of the affair for a considerable period of time, but had not raised it with her husband because she did not want a rift in the family. She had argued to herself that her husband was no less attentive to her than he had ever been, nor was he any less generous or caring. She had come to terms with the fact that if he needed this extra relationship, it was probably better all round if she turned a blind eye to it. Ellen's view of life was entirely different, since she was still idealistic enough to believe in 'happy ever after' families. Her grieving was very affected by the knowledge of her father's infidelity, since he now appeared to be a stranger to her rather than the father she had known and idolized.

A rather different problem confronted Maggie Williams. She had been married for 30 years when her husband died. They owned their own house and had lived reasonably comfortably, though her husband was constantly telling her to take care so that they did not get into financial difficulties. As a result, Mrs Williams had often gone without things that she needed in order that she could keep her children's standards up to that of their friends. When her husband's affairs were being put into order, it was discovered that in fact he was relatively rich, because he had been assiduously saving all their married life without telling his wife. The years of semi-deprivation had not been necessary.

ANGER

Finding that the person who has died was not in fact exactly the person that they were thought to be can cause enormous anger directed towards the deceased. Ellen (see under unexpected disclosures) was extraordinarily angry with her father. She felt that he was not the man she had believed him to be. She felt that he had taken enormous risks of hurting her mother and she also felt angry that he was no longer there for her to tell him just how cross and angry she was. Mrs Williams (see under unexpected disclosures) was also angry, not so much with her husband, but with the fact that he had not shared with her his need to build up a good financial background against whatever emergency he had been concerned might occur.

Sometimes this anger is deflected towards another person. For example, Ellen was also extremely angry with her father's mistress. She felt that this woman had somehow stolen something from the family by having this affair with her father. Such anger needs to be diffused, or it is liable to get in the way of the individual being able to grieve with normal parameters (Ch. 8).

JEALOUSY

Another emotion that can happen within a family after a death is jealousy, either jealousy of the siblings or other members of the family or, as in Ellen's situation, jealousy of an unknown person who had taken the love of her father that she felt had properly belonged to her mother and herself.

Arguments over the will

The jealousy may be triggered by the contents of the will. If one family member has been left something that another family member wanted, there is often very heated discussion and angry exchanges within a family. Joe Spiers had lived in the family home with his mother for all of his life. He was 35, he had not married and he looked after his mother in her final illness some years after his father had been killed in an accident.

When the will was read, Joe was left the contents of his mother's house. The house was to be sold and Joe and his two brothers would each receive one third of the selling price plus an equal share of their mother's other assets after bills had been settled. The brothers were very jealous that the family treasures had all been left to Joe. They forgot in their own grief and anger that he was the one member of the family who had cared and stayed with their frail mother. An enormous quarrel erupted weeks after the death when Joe offered to buy out his brothers' share of the house. The matter was eventually sorted out by the family solicitor and Joe was able to buy out his brothers' share. Family dynamics were very badly affected in this instance, by the jealousies and anger around the contents of the mother's will.

SHARED GRIEF

The ideal paradigm of family grief is that the death brings family members closer together and that they can share their sorrow. They can talk to each other about their feelings and discharge the many emotions that surround the death by talking about guilt, anger, blame and jealousy. They can reconvene as a family adapting to the loss of a much loved member.

The task for the health professional is to identify those families where grief is not shared, and particularly those family members who feel isolated from the others in their group. In identifying the family dynamics, it is usually possible to further identify those members of the family who need assessing for the way they are coping with their grief. In this way, the most vulnerable members may be identified and helped. It is important to remember that to offer to see the whole family together on a first visit will probably inhibit its members from discussing their true feelings. By identifying key family members and talking to them individually, it will be much more possible to build up a picture of any insoluble problems. This may then be the point at which to offer to see the relevant individuals together, if they feel they need help.

DIFFERENTIAL COPERS

Perhaps one of the most important elements in considering grief within the family is to acknowledge that family members will not all grieve in the same way. Some people find it easier to deal with a problem by talking about it and by working through what it is that is troubling them, and what they might be able to do to make it better. Other individuals tend to put things behind them and may not want to talk. They will often admit that talking is just too painful and that they would prefer to leave things alone. This may be a normal coping mechanism for them.

The problem in a family occurs when close family members cope in these different ways. The person who wants to talk is an irritant to the member who does not want to talk, and often feelings can run high because of these different methods of coping. Again this needs to be identified and addressed.

What is important here is that neither method of coping is more 'right' than another. The aim of the person who is helping the family is to help them to find bridges that allow each to understand the other while respecting their methods of coping (Faulkner 1992).

INVISIBLE GRIEVERS

The 'other woman'

Those who have the most difficulty in expressing their grief are often those who are not meant to be grieving. Ellen's father's mistress, for example, was a professional woman who had kept her affair very secret from colleagues and friends. She was not able to go to the family house and see the body. She did go to the funeral standing at the very back of the church so that nobody would see her, but was sad that she could not send flowers. She had no outlet for showing her grief, and became very quiet and introspective. Ellen would have argued that this was no more than she deserved, but eventually her father's mistress sought professional help, since she became disordered by her unexpressed grief and the attendant guilt of being 'the other woman'.

The ostracized member of the family

A similar situation can occur with a family member. James

Miller was the eldest son of a medical family. He was bright, did well at school and it was fully expected that he would go to university and follow in his father's footsteps, one day taking over his general practice. When James was 18 he met and fell in love with an Asian girl. The girlfriend was unacceptable to the family for a number of reasons; she was coloured and their middle-class background made it difficult for them to accept this; and she was seen to be a bad influence on their much-loved child who was about to go to university. His girlfriend's family also objected to James. James was insulted at the way that his girlfriend was perceived and ran off with her, finding a job, setting up home and cutting himself off from his family.

He did in fact keep in touch with the family through his younger brother who had been the one member to understand how James was feeling. As a result James heard when his mother was dying. He visited her at the hospice and while he was there having a very sensitive reunion with his mother, his father came in and ordered him out of the hospice. James was asked not to visit again, because it was too upsetting for everybody. Again he did not see the body, he was not allowed to go to the funeral, and he and his wife were ostracized. He felt unable to display his grief because he was made to feel that he had brought the problems on himself, and had contributed to his mother's death.

The bereavement visitor, when talking to family members a few weeks after the death, did not even realize that James existed. He, on the other hand, did not tell his colleagues and friends of what had happened, partly because he was ashamed of his runaway behaviour in earlier years, but secondly, because he was so angry that he felt he dare not let that anger out.

WORKING WITH THE FAMILY

Working with the family means working with those individuals within a family who may need help. They may need this on an individual basis; a spouse who has received help will then feel perhaps a little bit stronger so that he can support other family members. If, however, major problems are identified within the family that have been exacerbated by the death, it may be useful to suggest that the bereavement visitor meets the family, simply to help them to talk to each other. The role here is to facilitate family discussion and disclosure, and should only be done after individual assessment of the family members concerned. If the problems are so severe that therapy is required, then the family should be referred for family therapy, if they feel themselves that this would be of benefit to them.

What has to be remembered is that in the weeks following a death, emotions may still be quite high and individuals in their grief are unable to see logical conclusions to their problems. The family may need help in moving on from the 'if only' syndrome to realize that one cannot recast the past, but one can adapt to the present with all its difficulties.

SUMMARY

In this chapter it has been seen that:

- Grief within a family may mean many different things.
- That much will depend on the closeness of the dead person and the particular family member, along with the type of relationship and any long-standing problems that may have been present.
- Within the family there are many emotions that are inter-related with different family members. These may include guilt, blame, jealousy and anger.
- It cannot be assumed that family members will all cope in the same way with their grief, or that all family members will be free to show their grief.
- In identifying the particular family member's problems it should be possible to draw a conclusion as to whether the family will cope in its own way by supporting other family members, or whether the family may need someone to facilitate open dialogue so that grief can be expressed.
- In families where the grief is so disabling that family therapy is required, the family should, with their permission, be referred on.

REFERENCES

Faulkner A 1992 Effective interaction with patients. Churchill Livingstone, Edinburgh
Kubler Ross E 1972 On death and dying.

FURTHER READING

Keitner G L, Miller I W 1990 Family function and major depression: An overview. American Journal of Psychiatry, 147: 1128–1137.

8

The grieving child

When working with bereaved people, children in the family may often not be considered as part of the equation. It is often assumed, quite wrongly, that parents who are suffering bereavement themselves will be able to support and help their children. Further, children have often been excluded from the death or from knowledge of the death since many parents consider that their child would be best not to get involved. Secondly, it may be assumed that children do not understand a great deal about dying (Adams & Deveau 1984). In fact, quite young children have some concept of death as shown in the following example:

Mary and her granny were walking up the village on their way home from the hairdresser's.

Mary: 'Granny, stay on the path, it's dangerous on the road'.

Granny: 'Yes, we'll both stay on the pavement, Mary'.

Mary: 'If you went in the road you'd be run over by a car'.

Granny: 'That's right Mary, I might well'.

Mary: 'And if you were run over by a car you'd be dead'.

Granny: 'Oh gosh'.

Mary:	'Please don't worry granny. If you're dead in the road, I'll get the doctor'.
Granny:	'And what will the doctor say?'
Mary:	'The doctor will look at you granny and he'll say, "When you're dead, you can only get deader"'.

Mary was three when this interaction took place. What she showed was that she understood about accidents and death. She later in the same weekend showed that she didn't really understand causes of death.

Granny:	'Mary, what a pretty necklace'.
Mary's mum:	'Yes, don't you recognize it. It's one you gave me'.
Granny:	'Yes, it used to belong to my mother'.
Mary:	'Doesn't your Mummy want it any more, Granny?'
Granny:	'Well, my Mummy doesn't need it any more, she's dead'.
Mary:	'Did somebody shoot her?'

Some young children have some concept of the permanence of death. However, others do not, so in talking to a child about the concept it is necessary to find out just exactly what they think dying means. Those who are exposed to a lot of television where they see cartoon characters dead one minute and alive the next, may not quite grasp the permanence of death. Further, they may not entirely understand why people die. Neither of these facts should prevent parents and others who are in the child's family circle from trying to help the child to understand what death is all about.

PARENTS' REASONS FOR COLLUSION

In talking to parents, many of them feel that the death of someone that the child loves will cause extreme unhappiness. Because they love their children and want to protect them from pain, they may argue that the child does not need to know about the impending death until it has actually occurred. What many parents do not realize is that by excluding children from what is a family crisis, those children may later feel very bitter and resentful that they were not involved, and not trusted to understand what was happening in the family.

Duncan, aged 12, was being assessed to find out how much he knew about his mother's terminal illness. He had worked out that whatever was wrong with his mother must be 'pretty serious' because nobody was telling him anything. When asked how he felt about that, he said,

'They treat you like a screaming 2-year-old who doesn't have an intellect'(Help the Hospices 1992).

Parents may need to be helped to involve their children in the period before the death of the loved person in the child's life.

HELPING PARENTS TO INVOLVE CHILDREN

If parents discuss involving the children in an impending death, they often talk in very black and white terms (Help the Hospices 1992).

> Rob, whose wife was dying of breast cancer, did not want to involve his two children of 12 and 14, and argued that it was very difficult to talk to children about impending death.
>
> Nurse: 'So you can't think of any good reasons to tell the children what's going on?'
>
> Rob: 'Well, no. They know she's ill, but I can't say anything else than that. I could tell them that she's ill one day and next that she's very ill, and the next that she's very, very ill. There isn't much elasticity in "ill" '.

A model for involving children

What parents need very much is help in understanding how their children will approach the change in the family routine caused by the fact of the dying person and their needs. A model for involving children that seems to work very well is that of breaking bad news described by Faulkner (1992). The child is given the warning shot, i.e. that the person that they love is ill and won't be able to do the sort of things with the child that they have been used to doing. This is followed by giving information at the rate the child shows that it is ready to receive it (Table 8.1).

Table 8.1 Breaking bad news (adapted from Faulkner 1992)

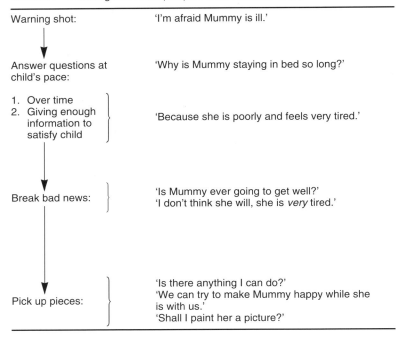

Warning shot:	'I'm afraid Mummy is ill.'
Answer questions at child's pace:	'Why is Mummy staying in bed so long?'
1. Over time 2. Giving enough information to satisfy child	'Because she is poorly and feels very tired.'
Break bad news:	'Is Mummy ever going to get well?' 'I don't think she will, she is *very* tired.'
Pick up pieces:	'Is there anything I can do?' 'We can try to make Mummy happy while she is with us.' 'Shall I paint her a picture?'

Some children may get quickly to the point and ask if Mummy or Granny is ever going to get better and then the bad news is broken, 'Well, no, I'm afraid that she isn't.' Other children will need the information in much slower stages, for example:

Monday

Susan, aged 8: 'Mummy, why hasn't Daddy gone to work today?'

Mummy: 'Because he's not very well, darling'.

Susan: 'Will he be able to take me to Brownies tonight?'

Mummy: 'No, don't worry about Brownies, darling, I'll take you there'.

Friday

Susan: 'Mummy, is daddy going to stay in bed all the time?'

Mummy: 'Well, no darling, he's not. In fact he's going to the hospital tomorrow'.

Susan: 'And will they make him better there?'

Mummy: 'They don't know yet'.

Susan continued asking her mother questions over a series of weeks until the day when she had obviously worked out what was going on.

Susan: 'Mummy?'

Mummy: 'Yes darling'.

Susan: 'They didn't make Daddy better at the hospital, did they?'

Mummy: 'No darling, they didn't'.

Susan: 'Does that mean that he'll never get better?'

Mummy: 'Come and give me a cuddle. I'm afraid you're right'.

Susan: 'Is Daddy going to Jesus?'

Mummy: 'Who told you that?'

Susan: 'My teacher at school in prayers today said we must all pray for my Daddy because he's going to Jesus'.

Mummy (somewhat taken aback):

          'Well, yes I'm afraid you're right. Daddy isn't going to get better. Shall we go and say hello to him now?'

Susan: 'Can I ask him about Jesus?'

Mummy: 'Well, let's just see how it goes, shall we?'

In this situation the child had gained the final understanding from her school, and this is a problem for many parents if the child gets information from outside the home. However, by involving Susan and answering her questions as they came, she adapted, albeit very sadly, to the fact that her Daddy was going away and that this time, unlike his previous business trips, he would not be coming back. Because Susan and her mother were both involved, their grieving was mutual and more manageable than if Susan had been excluded.

Some children do not ask questions and may not respond to a 'warning shot'. A parent or family friend can help here by checking out with the child.

Mother to children (9 & 11 years): 'I wanted to talk to you about Grannie. She isn't at all well'.

Sue (9):	'She is always in bed'.
Alan (11):	'That is because she is old—silly!'
Sue:	'I'm not silly'.
Mother:	'Come on! I'm afraid Grannie is tired *and* ill'.
Sue (sounding frightened):	'Will she die?'
Mother:	'I'm afraid she will darling'.
Alan:	'Why didn't she tell me?'
Sue:	'Or me?'
Mother:	'I'm afraid she is finding things difficult just now—but she may want to talk to us later. She certainly wants to see you'.
Sue:	'What can we take her?'

Often the child will appear to accept reality in a very pragmatic way initially, but come back to the subject later with more questions.

Parents with their own problems

Many parents argue that their child would not be able to adapt as Susan has done or to really understand what is going on, but if the information is given to the child as the child requests it, then little damage will be done, and mutual comfort can occur between parents and child. What is difficult is the fact that the parent who is facing the death of a partner or some other close family member has problems of their own, and this may make them less sensitive to their children's needs. This is where a close family member living nearby or a loving neighbour can help the child come to grips with the situation if the parent is having difficulty themselves.

Surprised by knowledge

Because death is a subject that is little talked about in western culture, many parents may be surprised by their children's knowledge of death. Very often a child in the class at school has been ill and thought to be in danger. Occasionally a child will learn about road traffic accidents and the fact that people can be killed on their way to school while feeling perfectly well. Similarly, they may have knowledge of death from reading, from talking to their peers, and from other media sources.

The advantages of involvement

By involving children in the reality of an impending death, there is the chance then for the child to tell the dying person how much they care about them, and to do things for them that will leave them memories of having helped. This is in stark contrast to the child who was not told that a much loved person is dying, and after the death felt that they perhaps could have helped more or done more, or made gifts for the dying person. No child should be denied this right.

THE PARENTS

Involving a child in an impending death can be very painful for the parent concerned. They may have to answer very difficult questions, some of which they are not sure how to answer. For example, the child who has been told that Daddy is going to Jesus may want a description of heaven and what goes on there. This has to be handled very carefully, so as not to give the child an unrealistic view of what has happened.

Box 8.1   A misleading approach

Danny was very close to his grandmother who died when he was five. He knew that Granny was very ill and he knew that one day she would go away. When he asked where she had gone after the death, he was told she had gone to live in Jesus' house. He seemed to accept this quite readily, though he did occasionally ask if granny would come back. He was told that, no, she was always going to live in Jesus' house now, but that she was happy and that she still loved him.

Everything was fine until Easter, when Danny's parents took him to a children's Easter service at the local church. Danny, who had been very good and very well behaved up until that moment, suddenly started rushing all over the church. As his mother tried to corner him and bring him back to the pew, she asked him what the trouble was. Danny burst into loud sobs,

'You said she was here, you said that Granny was in Jesus' house and I can't find her.'

The above example shows that the use of euphemisms to explain death must be considered very carefully, so that children do not get a wrong impression or unrealistic hopes about the re-emergence of the person that they love who has died.

By involving the child in the period before death, there is an opportunity for the child to actually be involved in the death itself. They may wish to say goodbye to the person whom they love and tell them how much they love them. It seems to be very important to children that they have such an opportunity. They may not know exactly when Granny is going to die, or when Daddy will die, but if adults take them to see the dying person a little while before the death, then the child should know that this may be their last opportunity to see their beloved relative. They may then feel free to talk to the dying person and give them loving messages. Again, the difficulties are often for the adult, not for the child, for example:

Simon (aged 10): 'Aunty Mabel, do you like it here in the hospice?'

Aunty Mabel: 'Well, they look after me very well dear'.

Simon: 'But you're not going to get better are you?'

Aunty Mabel: 'No darling, I'm not going to get better, but I'm glad you've come to see me'.

Simon: 'I've brought you a present'.

Aunty Mabel: 'What have you brought me?'

Simon: 'It's a biscuit. I made it myself'.

Simon didn't in fact say goodbye to Aunty Mabel, and Aunty Mabel was rather upset that he knew that she was going to die, but they left each other with love and happy memories. Simon still remembers making the biscuits and now he can laugh about whether anyone would have eaten the soggy offering, let alone a dying patient.

SEEING THE BODY

There are different opinions on whether children should see the body of a loved person or not. Some parents argue that it will upset the child, while others say that they know that it is good for the child to see the body in order to accept the death.

Box 8.2   A matter of choice

It is argued that seeing the body is a matter of choice for the child, as is attending the funeral. What is important is that that choice is made *by* the child and not *for* the child.

Children who do not wish to see a dead person and who do not wish to go to a funeral may be able to say their goodbyes in other ways. Kathy, who was 7, said she did not want to go to her Granny's funeral, but later came to her mother with a little envelope and said,

'I've written to Granny. I've written goodbye to Granny and told her I want her to be happy with Jesus. Will you take it with you when you go to the funeral?'

The child's pragmatism

One of the difficulties for parents when handling children and bereavement is the child's pragmatism.

David lived with his parents in a biggish old house that had a flat at the back in which his Granny lived. David and his Granny were very good friends. When he came home from school at night, he always went to say hello to Granny before going to his mother. When his Granny was ill, her bed was brought down from the flat into the dining room of David's home and every day when he came from school he would come and say hello to Granny.

Because Granny had lived near David for a long time they did lots of things together, and she had always promised David that when she did not need it any more, he would be able to have her tool set that she kept for minor jobs and also that he would be able to have the Lego castle that was kept for other visiting grandchildren. David's Granny died in the middle of the night and his mother was very concerned that David should not see her dead. The funeral directors came in the middle of the night to take the body away. The bed was subsequently dismantled and when David came down the next day, the dining room looked as it had before his Granny's illness.

David: 'Where's granny?'

Mummy: (crying)

David: 'Why are you crying? Did Granny die?'

Mummy: 'Yes, I'm afraid she did'.

David: 'Can I have the Lego castle now, then can I go and get the tool kit?'

With that, David rushed off and his mother became very angry that he was so uncaring. In fact David was lying on his bed sobbing his heart out an hour later, but his pragmatism simply allowed him to say out loud what many adults might have been thinking in terms of inheritance after a death.

A need for a framework

Children's need for information and their pragmatic approach to life may also bring difficult questions to parents.

Mandy knew that her uncle was dying and was quite upset about it. When she found out that he had died, she asked her own father what would happen to her dead uncle.

Father: 'Well Mandy, when somebody dies they don't need their body any more. The bit that we love and care about goes up to Heaven and then the body, which is now a shell, we have to dispose of it'.

Mandy: 'What do you mean, dispose?'

Father: 'Well, with Uncle Jack we're going to cremate him'.

Mandy: 'What's cremate?'

Father: 'Well, that bit of uncle that we don't need will be burnt'.

Mandy: 'Daddy?'

Father: 'Yes . .'

Mandy: 'Is this going to be one of your do-it-yourself bonfires?'

Again, her father was very upset, but this was Mandy trying to put a new concept into some sort of framework that she could understand.

This ability to talk, to ask questions, is very necessary if the child is going to cope with their grief, but it must be remembered that this constant need for talking and information from a child may cause the parents or loved ones who are also grieving considerable emotional pain. Not all children will want to talk. They may hug their grief to themselves and feel that it is too private and too painful to talk about. There is no way one can force a child to disclose how they are feeling, but they can be encouraged to talk when they feel inclined, and helped to express their feelings.

Differential copers

Too often there is the concern that all people should deal with their grief in the same way. This is as variable in children as it is in adults. It can be a problem if siblings cope in a different way, and then the children might well start falling out with each other. If, for example, one child wants to talk and the other does not, the child who does want to talk may start attacking the child who does not. Parents in this situation need to intervene without appearing to take sides, perhaps explaining gently to both children that people deal with problems in different ways, that it is all right to talk, but that it is equally all right not to talk if that seems to be the best way forward for that person.

Time is important here, for where some children are prepared to express their grief soon after the death, other children may need a little longer before they feel safe enough to express their feelings. Those children may express their grief in different ways but when asked might say something to the effect that it hurts too much to talk about the feelings.

ASSESSING A BEREAVED CHILD

Assessing a bereaved child should follow a very similar pattern to assessing an adult. The child should be given the opportunity to talk and helped to talk about the same areas as an adult. Did they go to the funeral? How did they feel when they knew when their loved person was dead?

In many ways, assessing a bereaved child is easier than an adult because children, on the whole, have not learnt to put up the social barriers that cover feelings. The first experience of death that a child may have may be the loss of a much loved pet and even here the child is able, at quite an early age, to talk about what it was like for them.

Mary (aged 4):	'My doggy died. Merlin died'.
Neighbour:	'How did Merlin die?'
Mary:	'He ran into the road'.
Neighbour:	'And what did you think of that Mary?'
Mary:	'I cried. Mummy said did I want to see Merlin'.
Neighbour:	'Did you see him?'
Mary:	'Yes. He looked all right, but he wasn't moving'.
Neighbour:	'What else did you notice?'
Mary:	'His fur was soft like it's always soft. I asked him to wake up'.
Neighbour:	'And what happened then?'
Mary:	'He wouldn't. I cried. I made his fur wet. Mummy said I should come away but Daddy said if I liked I could see them put Merlin somewhere safe'.
Neighbour:	'And where was that?'
Mary:	'It was in the garden by the big tree. Daddy digged a hole'.
Neighbour:	'And did you stay there?'
Mary:	'Yes. I was sitting on the ground touching Merlin'.
Neighbour:	'And what happened when Daddy had dug the hole?'
Mary:	'I helped Mummy and Daddy to lay him in the hole. We put his blanket in the hole and then he laid on his blanket'.
Neighbour:	'What else happened?'
Mary:	'I asked if I could put some food in for him'.
Neighbour:	'And did you?'
Mary:	'No. Mummy said he wouldn't need it any more'.

In the above sequence it can be seen that Mary was very involved in the death of her pet. She saw the body, she touched him, she saw him buried, and she even thought of trying to equip him to be there on his own. Her parents attempted to maintain a sense of reality although they conceded and put the blanket in the hole. They explained to Mary that the dog would not need food to help her accept that Merlin was dead.

This early experience helped Mary considerably when later a school friend was killed and she had to hear about it and try to make sense of what had happened. In assessing a child, it is very important to use language that makes sense to the child and then to ask questions in a simple way. This gives the child the opportunity to talk about their feelings and what sense they are making of the current situation.

Often the child will talk about the dead person in terms of where they have gone. They seem less able than an adult to understand the finality of death and so they may need to talk through hopes and fears and be gently corrected if they have an unreal expectation.

Martin:	'Who are you?'
Bereavement Volunteer:	'Well I'm the lady who comes to talk to people when somebody they love has died. I thought it might be nice if I could talk to you'.
Martin:	'What do you want to talk about?'
Volunteer:	'I want to know how you feel now that Mummy died'.
Martin:	'I don't know'.
Volunteer:	'Well, can you tell me something about what happened to Mummy'.
Martin:	'Well she got ill. Her face went all yellow and she was thin and then she stayed in bed a lot, and Daddy didn't go to work'.
Volunteer:	'And what was happening to you then?'
Martin:	'Well, I went to school. Daddy looked after us but he was often cross'.
Volunteer:	'What happened then?'
Martin:	'One day when I came in from school, Daddy said Mummy had gone away'.

Volunteer:	'And where had she gone to?'
Martin:	'She'd gone to Heaven. We all went to church to say goodbye to her'.
Volunteer:	'How did you feel?'
Martin:	'I just wish she'd come back'.

EMOTIONAL REACTIONS

Emotional reactions in children are very similar to those of adults. They are often confused and worried, upset, maybe angry with the dead person for going away, sometimes angry with the surviving relative who is there, often very guilty indeed for imagined wrongs that they have done to the dead person, and this particularly happens if a parent has threatened a child over good behaviour.

Michael, aged 10, was quite convinced that his mother had died because of his poor behaviour simply because when she got cross with him, when she was well, she used to say,

'If you don't behave, you'll be the death of me.'

These feelings and beliefs need to be assessed and brought into the open, so that the child has a chance to talk through their feelings and to reach some realization that they were not in any way responsible for what happened to their dead parent.

Handling the emotions of children is similar to handling those of adults. Anger needs to be expressed, diffused, and accurately focused.

Michael:	'I didn't know Mummy would really die'.
Visitor:	'And how does that leave you feeling?'
Michael:	'Cross'.
Visitor:	'Cross?'
Michael:	'Yes, cross with her for going—she knew I didn't mean to be naughty' (beginning to cry).
Visitor:	'Sounds like you think you sent her away'.
Michael:	'She always said I'd be the death of her'.
Visitor:	'And do you believe that?'

Michael (hesitating):	'I'm not sure'.

Further work with Michael helped him to deal with his anger and guilt, though he maintained some belief that things may have been different if he could have foreseen his mother's death.

A problem for children in sharing their feelings within the family is the level of grief in their carers, but if they have been involved in reality before the death they appear to cope better afterwards since they feel as equally involved as other family members.

SUMMARY

Children are often excluded from the impending death of somebody close to them whom they love:

- They may be denied the right to see the dead body, to say goodbye or to attend the funeral.
- Parents need help in involving their children, realizing that this is going to be good in the long term.
- By protecting the child today, they may be causing problems in the future.
- Children who are at risk of not coping with their grief should be assessed in the same way as adults.
- They should be encouraged to talk about the time around the death, the events following, and to discuss their feelings and their emotional reactions.
- If children and parents can talk to each other at the time of grief, then there are less likely to be problems for the future.

REFERENCES

Adams and Deveau 1984
Help the Hospices 1992 Child of a dying parent (video). Screen Productions, London

BOOKS FOR CHILDREN

Burningham J 1989 Granpa. Jonathan Cape, London
Buchanon Smith D 1987 A taste of blackberries. Puffin, London

Couldrick A 1990 Mum or Dad has cancer. Sobell, Oxford
Kopper L 1982 When Uncle Bob died. Dinosaur, Cambridge
Little J 1986 Mamma's going to buy you a mocking bird. Penguin, London
Mellonie B, Ingpen R 1983 Beginnings and endings with lifetimes in between.
   Dragons World, Surrey
Sims A 1986 Am I still a sister? Big A, New York
Stickney D 1984 Waterbugs and dragonflies. Mowbray, London
Varley S 1985 Badger's parting gifts. Picture Books. Collins, London

Bereavement visiting

Many bereaved people may only need one assessment visit. The visitor will find that this person, although probably still very sad and upset by the death of a loved one, is nevertheless coping reasonably well. That person may also have good support from family and friends and be seen to be managing to get back to some semblance of normal life.

Some people, however, may need further support. In the first assessment, the visitor will have realized that this person, although beginning to talk about feelings and about the loss of a loved one, may be in need of further help. The visitor will have asked herself the question,

'Can I help this individual to get in touch with her feelings and work through her grief, or do I need to refer this person to more specialist help than I can give?'

NEGOTIATION

If, at the end of an assessment, the visitor decides that a bereaved person may need more help, this should be negotiated as follows:

Visitor: 'Mrs Smith, I can see that things have been very difficult for you since the death of your husband, and although you do seem to be getting on quite well, I wonder if it would help you if I were to come and see you, much as I've seen you today, for a few more times?'

Mrs Smith: 'I'm not sure'.

Visitor: 'Not sure?'

Mrs Smith: 'Well, it's been good of you to come today, but it's brought it all back and I think I feel pretty sad at the moment. I don't know if I want to go on doing that'.

Visitor: 'Well, I can see how sad you are. Can you think of any benefit of having talked to me today?'

Mrs Smith: 'Well, before you came it was all bottled up. I didn't realize it would be so painful letting it out'.

Visitor: 'And it sounds as if you don't want to risk that pain in future'.

Mrs Smith: 'I'm just not sure'.

In the above exchange the visitor had quite correctly identified that Mrs Smith needed more time to work through her pain. Mrs Smith, however, was not sure that she was ready at that time, but as a result of that negotiation, she undertook to ring the bereavement visitor in 2 weeks' time to tell her how she was feeling. In fact Mrs Smith phoned slightly sooner, to say that, in retrospect, it had helped her to talk and she would like the visitor to come back. The decision had to be Mrs Smith's, but when that decision had been made, the visitor contracted further visits.

Mrs Smith was slightly ambivalent about further bereavement visits and needed time to consider risks and benefits. The opposite can occur in that some bereaved people are anxious for regular contact with the bereavement visitor, for example:

Visitor: 'Well Jane, thank you for talking to me today. I wonder though if it would help you if I were to come again'.

Jane: 'Oh, yes please, it's been so good to have somebody who lets me talk'.

Visitor: 'Well, shall we say that I'll come back again in 2 weeks' time?'

Jane: 'No, no, I'd like you to come next week if you possibly can'.

In the above sequence, the visitor had to negotiate with Jane on timing and find the time that was both possible for the visitor and of maximum benefit to Jane.

CONTRACTING

Contracting sounds quite a hard term for arranging to meet and talk with people who are suffering the loss of somebody that they love dearly. However, it is important that some form of contract is made so that both the visitor and the bereaved person have a clear idea of the frequency of visits, and how many visits might occur. It is often argued that in contracting, the bereavement visitor is in fact rationing time and giving a message that they do not want to spend too much time with the bereaved person. In fact, the opposite is true. What the bereavement visitor is saying is a good news message:

'You will not always need me'.

If the message is put in a positive way then the bereaved person is unlikely to believe that they are being a burden to the visitor, for example:

Visitor: 'Jane, I think it's going to be a bit too often if I come every week. Let's say that I come once every 2 weeks and we'll review the situation after a couple of months'.

Jane: 'A couple of months? That doesn't sound very long'.

Visitor: 'Well, we'll review it then. Maybe by then you might benefit from further visits, but they may not need to be so often, and if you are doing really well you may be able to cope on your own after that'.

Jane: 'Gosh, I'd like to think that that would be possible'.

In the above exchange, Jane could see that there was a positive message in contracting, though she remained doubtful whether the positive outcome of coping on her own after 2 months was possible.

TIME

Just as the time spent on the assessment visit (Ch. 5) should be negotiated, so should the time spent on follow-up visits. This again is beneficial to both the visitor and the bereaved individual. If the bereaved person knows when the visitor is coming and how long they are likely to be, then they can organize the rest of their life and concentrate on the visitor when she comes, rather than worrying about how long she may stay, and whether it will conflict with other priorities such as collecting children from school.

This has a double benefit, for talking about the bereavement may be very painful indeed, and the individual may benefit from knowing that any pain they experience in talking about the person they loved will be relatively short-lived. Half an hour (a reasonable time for a bereavement visit) can seem very long indeed, and certainly is long enough to go through the talking required on the areas of concern for the bereaved person.

PURPOSE

The purpose of follow-up visits should be clearly negotiated. The assessment visit has a purpose of identifying whether the patient is coping with their bereavement, whether they need further help, or whether they are so disordered that they need to be referred on elsewhere. The follow-up visit should be for those individuals who are not coping tremendously well with the death of their loved one, but who certainly do not need further specialist help.

In the assessment visit, areas of difficulty will have been identified and these should be the object of follow-up visits. This will allow further exploration of areas of difficulty and hopefully allow the person to work towards solutions that will help them in their adaptation to the death of the loved person.

Moving on

When Mr Blake (Ch. 5) was treated for his clinical depression following his wife's death, he was referred to the bereavement visitor for further work. The areas that he needed to cover were related to his actually accepting how life could possibly go on without his wife. This meant reviewing the way that things were when his wife was alive, looking at areas where the relationship was very dependent and also working on areas where Mr Blake had had hobbies that were his and which included his friends.

By helping Mr Blake to work through these areas, he himself began to make plans to re-open hobbies and friendships and also to seek other company to fill the gaps left by his wife. In this he did not want a new relationship. He was not yet ready for that, but what he did want was the company of other people.

Because bereavement visiting is painful both for the bereaved person and the visitor, there is a risk that the sessions can turn into cosy tea and chat. This leaves both people feeling quite comfortable but it does not deal with the problems with which the bereaved individual is grappling. Consider the two following interactions:

Mr Blake: 'Oh, nurse, it is good to see you'.

Visitor: 'It's good to see you too, Mr Blake. May I come in?'

Mr Blake: 'Oh yes, shall I make some tea? I've got some of those biscuits that you liked so much last time'.

Visitor: 'That's very kind of you. Where did you say you get them from?'

AND

Mr Blake: 'Oh nurse, it's so good to see you'.

Visitor: 'Well it's nice to see you looking a bit better. May I come in?'

Mr Blake: 'Shall I make some tea?'

Visitor: 'Let's do that later. First I'd like to ask you how you are getting on and talk through some of the areas that we agreed on last time'.

In the above sequences, the first is very likely to be social for perhaps half the time that the visitor has allowed, whereas in the second interaction the visitor firmly, but in a friendly way, made clear the purpose of her visit and agreed it with Mr Blake. One of the problems here is that the very people who need bereavement visits are often the people who need company as well, and they may often try to combine the visit with friendship which means that time is going to be difficult. Also, the purpose of the visit can be skewed by the social overtones that have been brought in at the beginning.

Changing purpose

Although the purpose of each visit may be set out on a previous occasion as with Mr Blake above, sometimes there are reasons why the purpose should change.

> Mrs Mason, a single parent whose child had died, had agreed to bereavement visits to talk through how she felt about the loss, and how she was coming to terms with the senselessness of it all. She had a boyfriend, but they did not live together. On the previous visit it had been agreed between them that the single mum would talk about how she had felt when she first knew her child was ill. She felt there was some unfinished business there and she wanted to talk through it to try to assuage some of the guilt that she felt at not noticing early enough that the child's pleas to stay away from school were perfectly legitimate.
>
> On the second visit, Mrs Mason met the visitor at the door.
>
> Visitor: 'Hello'.
>
> Mrs Mason: 'Come in, come in'.
>
> Visitor: 'You look very upset'.
>
> Mrs Mason: 'I am upset. I'm pregnant'.
>
> Later, when the visitor was settled in Mrs Mason's living room, Mrs Mason confided that she was having enormous problems in accepting the pregnancy. She loved her boyfriend and they had been talking of moving in together, but with her upset at the loss of her child she had put everything on hold. She now had to work through whether she wanted this new baby, and how that pregnancy was affected by her grief over the loss of her first child.

The above is a fairly unusual sequence of events, but in no way should the visitor on that occasion have said,
'Well, actually the purpose of my visit was for you to talk about your guilt'.
She had to go with the more important problem that Mrs Mason was dealing with on that day.

RE-ASSESSMENT

It is useful at the end of each bereavement visit to summarize the areas that have been covered and the work that has been done by the bereaved person. This allows negotiation to take place about further visits, but it also allows for regular re-assessment of the situation. Since the aim of the visit is to help people to move on through their grief, it is useful to discuss with the person from time to time how they feel they are progressing. This allows for renegotiation of the times and the frequency of the visits, as follows:

Visitor:	'Well, Mr Blake, I've seen you every 2 weeks over the last 2 months, and it seems to me from what you are saying that, although things are still pretty tough, they are getting easier. You've taken up the clay pigeon shooting again and you are enjoying that, and I see that you go down to the pub on Friday nights with Joe the way you used to. I know you've joined the Over-60s Club, though I'm not too sure how you feel about that yet'.
Mr Blake:	'Well, I suppose I'm finding my way in really. They are nice people but I'm not sure that I'm a "group" person'.
Visitor:	'Well, that's something we can talk about another time, and you're right, everybody doesn't respond well to group meetings'.
Mr Blake:	'You said that you'd come for the 2 months and that's up now. Are you going to leave me?'
Visitor:	'No, that's one of the things I wanted to talk to you about. It seems to me that things are better for you, but I feel that you've still got some way to go. I wondered if we could extend the time now, so that instead of coming every 2 weeks, I come every 3, and we'll review that in another month or so. It may be by then that you really don't need me any more'.
Mr Blake:	'That would be a really good news situation, wouldn't it? Sorry, I didn't mean to be rude'.
Visitor (laughing):	'You're not being rude, that's what we aim for, that after a while you won't need us any more'.

In the above exchange, Mr Blake was showing a readiness to consider life without the bereavement visitor and also to assess his own progress from suicidal beliefs after his wife's death, through to the treatment of his depression, and the picking up of some of the threads of his former life. He agreed readily to a new contract that was the beginning of tailing off the bereavement visits.

Further help

All bereavement visiting does not go so smoothly.

Jane, who had first of all wanted weekly visits, although accepting that they would in fact be fortnightly, always tried to extend the time that the visitor spent with her and several times asked that more frequent visits should take place. In this instance, when each session was reviewed and summarized, one of the areas that she had to deal with was Jane's excessive needs from her as an individual.

In re-assessing the situation, the visitor made this quite clear to Jane as follows:

Visitor: 'Well Jane, I've been visiting you now for 2 months, and this is the time we need to review. You seem to still be as needful of my visits as you were at the beginning, and this is something I think we should discuss next time I come. What I would like you to do between now and then, is to think of other opportunities for you to be social because I'm afraid that you appear to be turning me into a social friend rather than someone who is trying to help you with your grief. We need to consider ways forward that will expand your social life'.

Jane: 'But you're the only person who understands me. Nobody else wants me to talk about the death and what went on around it, just you'.

Visitor: 'Well, and that's another thing that we need to talk about, because you will reach a day when you can move on and need to talk less about the death. If when I see you next time we agree that that's not possible, it may be that you need to see somebody more experienced than myself to help you with this'.

In the above exchange, the visitor was putting it to Jane that she may need further help with her grief. Jane readily agreed to that, because she had insight into the fact that she needed to talk much more than anyone other than the bereavement visitor would currently allow her. This illustrates the fact that the decision to refer on may not always be made after the first assessment visit.

Managing on their own

Very often, on the date agreed for review, the visitor may feel that the bereaved person could now manage on their own. This has to be very carefully negotiated, because the individual may be a little nervous of giving up the help and support of the bereavement visitor.

Visitor:	'Mr Hurd, in the time that I've been visiting you, I've been really pleased to see how you've begun to adapt to the death of your wife. I can see that you're still very sad, but I get the impression that you seem to be managing your life in a more positive way'.
Mr Hurd:	'Oh yes, yes, in the early days it was just hell, but now, as you know, I'm beginning to get on with life again, though I do miss her'.
Visitor:	'And you will, but what I'm thinking about is the arrangement we made that I would see you until today, when we would review the situation. I'm wondering now if you are ready to go it alone'.
Mr Hurd:	'I don't know. Lots of the time now I think that I'm OK and that I can cope with it, but then there are the bad days still'.
Visitor:	'When did you last have a bad day?'
Mr Hurd:	'Well, it was just after you left last time. I went down the allotment, and the first of the peas were ready to pick. I started picking them, and then I went into my little shed down there to get the old colander, and suddenly it hit me that this year the new peas weren't something to surprise her with'.

Visitor:	'That must have been very hard'.
Mr Hurd:	'Yes. Yes, I did pick the peas and I put them in the colander and I went home. I gave them to my neighbour. I didn't think I could eat them on my own'.
Visitor:	'Well, how's it been since then?'
Mr Hurd:	'Oh, a few days later when I was down the allotment I could see that there was a second picking, and I just picked them. It was the first time that was so hard, but I could eat the second lot'.
Visitor:	'And that must tell you how well you are doing'.
Mr Hurd:	'Yes, I suppose it does'.
Visitor:	'You seem a little nervous about giving up these visits, so what I'd like to suggest is that we agree to stop them, but if you get a very bad day and you need someone to talk to, you can give me a ring. How's that?'
Mr Hurd:	'Well, I think that would be a bit like a comfort blanket if you didn't mind. I don't want to disturb you at home'.
Visitor (laughing):	'Oh, it's not my home number. This is the number of my office and if I'm not there, my secretary will know where to find me'.
Mr Hurd:	'You know it's meant a lot to me having someone listen and help me through'.
Visitor:	'Well, I'm pleased that it's worked for you'.

A telephone contact

Some bereaved individuals do not agree as readily as Mr Hurd, and one of the ways to deal with that is to lengthen the gap between meetings and tail them off in the same way as with Jane (p. 120). What a bereavement visitor will be looking for at the time of renegotiation, is that some strands of a normal life have been picked up, and some friendships renewed. The person may be more able to talk about their loved one than they were in the beginning, and to think more positively about their future. Eventually the bereaved individual should need no more than a telephone contact number that they can use if they really do feel concerned or overly upset at any time. Few people will use this number, but they find it a comfort and few will abuse the privilege, if the visitor has correctly assessed the stage of grieving that the individual has reached.

SUMMARY

In this chapter bereavement visits have been considered in the following ways:

- Whether they are necessary and how long they may be necessary for.
- The importance of negotiation in terms of setting a contract with the bereaved individual, so that they are quite clear about how often the visitor will come, what sort of time will be spent and what purpose the visits are going to fulfil.
- The significance of re-assessment as an ongoing activity, so that when the review date of the contract comes, the visitor and the bereaved person will themselves be able to agree whether the grief is well on its way.
- Hence they need to decide whether in fact they need to continue with visits, or whether the grief is not moving on and may need referring on to someone more specialized.
- The way in which negotiation takes place for a renewal of the contract, perhaps with larger gaps between the visits, or whether referral is necessary, have been demonstrated.
- Finally, suggestions have been made as to how to terminate visits while still leaving the lifeline of an office telephone number.

Letting go: potential problems

Unfortunately, bereavement visiting does not always follow the relatively smooth path described in chapter 9. Problems can arise when:

1. bereaved people demand more than the visitor should give, and
2. when the visitor gives more than is reasonable.

Either of these events can lead to a skewing of the bereavement visitor/individual relationship and if the problems are not identified and dealt with, can lead to misunderstandings and further grief for those who are bereaved.

DEPENDENCY

Dependency is a very common problem in bereavement work. The visitor is perceived as someone who will listen and help the person to work through their grief. In fact, the visit may be the high spot of the bereaved person's week if they are lonely and unhappy. Signs of this may emerge very early in the relationship, with the visitor noting that special cakes have been made or bought to be served, or other favourite foods of the visitor have been identified and supplied. The visit then becomes more like an afternoon tea party than a professional visit to someone who needs help.

The bereavement visitor may take such efforts as a sign of feedback that they are doing a good job and because they are flattered by the attention, they often neglect to note that these are the early signs of dependency.

Friendliness, not friendship

There are several dangers in dependency, firstly to the bereaved individual themselves, because, as inevitably happens, the bereavement visitor pulls out, then the bereaved person is in effect suffering a second loss. Secondly, if the dependency is not identified and curtailed early, the bereavement visitor is, albeit unconsciously, educating the person that it is acceptable to be dependent. This then raises the possibility of the bereaved individual feeling very bitter when the bereavement visitor eventually withdraws, for example:

Visitor: 'Jane, a few weeks ago we talked about how things were going, and I did suggest to you that you needed more specialist help'.

Jane: 'Well, yes, and I agreed to that, you know I did. I want to get better, I really do, but you'll still come, won't you?'

Visitor: 'Well, no. If I refer you on you won't need to see both of us'.

Jane: 'But I thought you were my friend'.

Visitor: 'No Jane, never your friend. I feel friendly towards you but my role in your life has been very much a helping one'.

Jane: 'Oh, you're just like everybody else. Everybody lets me down'.

In the above exchange it can be seen that Jane had misinterpreted her relationship with the bereavement visitor, and although she had the insight to see that she needed more specialist help, she had wanted to retain the visitor as a friend.

Pulling out

Another problem with dependency is for the visitor themselves, who may feel caught up in a situation where they cannot withdraw. It is not unusual for people to be visiting for long periods of up to 2 years or beyond after the death, when in reality visits should either have been terminated or, if the patient is in real need, they should have been referred on for more specialist help.

Another problem which is not often considered is that if a bereaved person becomes too dependent on their visitor, this may exclude the family and social circle that could support a person in their grief. Because the visitor is coming regularly and because the bereaved person finds that useful and rewarding, the rest of the family may withdraw from the difficult arena of bereavement, and even become less supportive than before the death.

Whose needs?

If a bereavement visitor finds that dependency is occurring, then there is an immediate need to re-assess the situation in terms of why it is arising and to give serious thought as to what can be done to bring the relationship back to the helping interaction that had been contracted with the bereaved person.

In many instances, dependency arises because the bereavement visitor is almost too good at meeting the needs of the individual concerned. It was seen with Jane that this was the one person whom she felt understood her and who was prepared to listen to her. Naturally, she did not want to give up this facility, and had not herself realized how dependent she had become on the kindly visitor who gave her full attention and encouraged her to talk about her grief.

When the bereavement visitor re-assessed the situation with Jane, she realized that she needed more specialist input than she could offer, but she also had to face the fact that she had allowed this client to become very dependent. This led to some heart-searching as to why this had occurred.

Encouraging dependency

Such introspection can be very painful, for often it reveals that the client is in fact meeting some need in the bereavement visitor. With hindsight, the visitor may realize that she had actually encouraged the dependency. Jane's visitor was relatively lonely. Although she worked full time, she also did voluntary work in the evenings and was very flattered by clients like Jane who made a special effort to provide refreshments and a comfortable setting. With the added incentive of feeling needed she had fallen into the trap of allowing dependency to occur.

Interdependence

In making the break with Jane, the visitor admitted that the interdependence had been probably quite useful to them both for a limited period, but now it was time for Jane to move on to more specialist help, and for the visitor to move on to newly bereaved people who also needed her help. The painful interview that ensued acted as a reminder when negotiating with other people who needed her help. In such situations it is really important to be honest with oneself, for it is too easy to blame a client for becoming too dependent, when in reality that dependency could not occur if proper ground rules had been set.

TRANSFERENCE

Newly bereaved people are very vulnerable and are facing life with a big gap left by the person whom they loved. Some actively seek to fill the gap while others, at an unconscious level, appear to be searching for someone who will take the place of their loved one. The bereavement visitor is at risk of being transferred into the place of the dead person, as are family members. As with dependence, this transference (Faulkner & Maguire 1994) needs to be recognized sooner rather than later.

Transference of a role

All transference is not so dramatic, and sometimes family responses encourage transference unwittingly. After a death, a small boy may be told,

'You have to be the daddy of the family now' or a girl may be told,

'You've got to be mummy to us all now'.

This is usually said in an attempt to comfort a newly bereaved child and give them a role in a family that is missing one of its most important members. However, it can lead to enormous problems as children try to fulfil roles for which they are not ready.

Box 10.1   The visitor as a replacement

Alice was working as a nurse at the local hospice when she met the Wheeler family. Mrs Wheeler had breast cancer with secondaries in her spine, and was dying. She was about the same age as Alice. Mr Wheeler was a pleasant, though rather confused, young man. He had two small children, did not understand why his wife was so ill at so young an age, and often stopped to talk to Alice when he visited his wife.

Alice could identify with this family. She became quite fond of Mrs Wheeler and felt that she knew the family well. At the point of Mrs Wheeler dying, Alice gave Mr Wheeler a big hug and said,
   'It must be terrible for you but we will be there to support you'.
She later offered to visit Mr Wheeler to see how he was coping. His mother was looking after the children, and he had returned to work and was trying to put his life back together. He was very grateful to Alice for the chance to talk through his thoughts and worries and actively looked forward to her fortnightly visits.

Alice found the visits quite rewarding as she watched Mr Wheeler move from being absolutely desolated to making some plans for his own and his children's future. Because Mr Wheeler worked, he asked if Alice could make her visits in the evenings so she generally went to the house at about 6 o'clock.

One evening Mr Wheeler asked her if the following week she could come a little later. She agreed to this, and was quite upset when she got to the house. The door was opened and over Mr Wheeler's shoulder she saw a candlelit table and heard soft music in the background. Suddenly Alice realized that Mr Wheeler was wanting her to have the sort of relationship that he had had with his wife. She admits that she took one look, took tail and ran.

What Alice had not recognized was that transference had taken place when she visited Mr Wheeler to talk to him about his grief.

Observing the ground rules

The beginning of transference can be recognized, though it is not always obvious. When Alice reviewed the situation that had led up to Mr Wheeler setting up a dinner for two, she thought of the number of visits she had made and how they had differed. The problem was that they had differed in such a small and subtle way that she had simply not been alert to what was happening. The first assessment visit was made and a contract was set that she would visit every fortnight for 2 months and then see how things were. On the second visit Mr Wheeler started to talk about his wife and their life together, and began to work through some of the pain of her death. After that the discussions had moved subtly to Mr Wheeler making allusions to similarities between Alice and his wife. This might take the form of noting that Alice was the same age as his wife or something to do with her physical appearance—both had been blonde.

This can act as a reminder that there is a purpose and a format to bereavement visiting with clear ground rules that should be observed when helping a person to work through some of the problems that they have in adjusting to the death of a loved one and to talk through their feelings. Observe the following interactions:

Mr Wheeler: 'I miss her so much, she was only 28. That must be about your age'.

Alice: 'That's clever. Yes, I was 28 two months ago'.

Mr Wheeler: 'Only 2 months ago, so you must be a Cancer subject too'.

AND

Mr Wheeler: 'I miss her so much, she was only 28. That must be about your age'.

Alice: 'Yes. Tell me what it is you miss about her so much'.

In the first exchange, Mr Wheeler began to make a personal comment about Alice to which she responded and thus allowed the conversation to develop at a personal level. In the second interaction, Alice nipped in the bud any chance of talking about her own age and kept the interaction very much on the topic for which she was there—

'Tell me why you miss your wife so much?'

This may seem hard, but it is even harder if transference is allowed to develop, for then the disengagement of the visitor from the bereaved person becomes yet another loss and disappointment to bear.

HELPING VERSUS BEFRIENDING

Those who visit the bereaved in a helping capacity often find themselves drawn into a friendship, and many would argue that this is all right, that the bereaved individual needs a friend as well as help in adapting to the death of their loved one. This can pose many problems, not least the cost to the bereavement visitor, who will have to set a limit on how many dependent friends they can have. Certainly those who visit the bereaved should be friendly but this is very different to being open to a friendship.

As with transference, friendship may creep into the relationship slowly and insidiously, so the visitor should be alert to the signs that what the bereaved person wants from them is more than a fortnightly visit to talk about the adaptation to loss, for example:

Visitor: 'Hello Avril, can I come in? What beautiful music you are playing'.

Avril: 'Yes, it's the Palestrina Masses. I love early Church music'.

Visitor: 'So do, I but I don't have that one'.

Avril: 'I could copy it on to a tape for you if you like'.

Visitor: 'Thanks, that would be lovely'.

Avril: 'OK. Now let me make some tea, it is good to see you'.

Many people would argue that the above sequence was no more than 'building a relationship' and some people really believe that it is not possible to talk about painful subjects until such niceties are over. However, if one looks more carefully at the interaction, it is very much an early friendship interaction with the common love of music as a starting point. From this can stem other commonalities so that eventually the visitor is no longer perceived as a bereavement visitor, but a friend. She may still have a helping role in the friendship, but it is no longer a contracted helping relationship that will start at a time of need and terminate when that need is lessened. The responsibility rests clearly with the visitor to maintain her role in a pleasant way which is friendly but which does not invite friendship, for example:

Visitor: 'Hello Avril, may I come in. What beautiful music'.

Avril: 'Yes, it's the Palestrina Masses. I love early Church music'.

Visitor: 'It's nice to see that you're listening to music again. How have things been in other respects?'

In the above, the visitor still disclosed her own appreciation of the music, but rather than developing that, as one would in a friendship, she brings it back to the purpose of her visit. This is not unfriendly but it is simply staying with a professional agenda rather than a personal one.

BOUNDARIES

It can be seen that to avoid the potential problems in bereavement work, one has to set boundaries. These boundaries can be spelt out to the bereaved individual at the beginning of the contract, not in a prescriptive way, but rather as an explanation about what bereavement visiting is all about and what the purpose of bereavement visits are.

Being honest

A main component of setting boundaries is an ability to be honest with the grieving person. If, for example, it is noted that dependency is arising, then this should be clearly stated. It might be, for example, that someone begins to say,

'I really look forward to your visits'.

Rather than being flattered by this growing need there is a requirement to explain that this is not what bereavement visiting is about, for example:

Jack:	'Do you know love, you're the most cheerful person I see these days. I really look forward to your visits'.
Visitor:	'That's nice Jack, but you mustn't get too dependent you know. I'm here to help you, but there are other people out there for you as well'.
Jack:	'Well, they're not very busy coming forward'.
Visitor:	'Well, perhaps we should talk about you going out to meet them half way'.
Jack (laughing):	'You mean perhaps I should start going to the pub again'.
Visitor:	'Well, would that be all bad?'

In the above exchange which was very friendly, the visitor points out that it would not be a good thing for Jack to become too dependent. His response tells her that he has taken this well. Agreeing a contract with the bereaved person and stating the time limits within that contract will also help to avoid the problems inherent in visiting someone who is vulnerable and in great need of much more than the bereavement visitor should be offering.

Boundaries on scope

Boundaries also need to be set on the scope of the work that the couple will do together. For example, death comes as a great shock to people who love the dead person, but it is easy to believe that their life was perfect prior to the death. In fact, most families have multiple problems that have been on-going for a number of years, and there is a need to differentiate with the bereaved individual the difference between long on-going family sagas and the problems arising as a result of the death of a loved one.

If this boundary is not set, the bereavement visitor can find themselves drawn in to all sorts of long-standing family problems that no-one else has solved for 20 years, and certainly should not be expected to be solved by the bereavement visitor.

To avoid a grieving person bringing in all their old family problems, it is important that clear guidelines are set on what areas are going to be covered.

Jack: 'Life would be easier if it wasn't for the problem with my sister and her husband'.

Visitor: 'Has that happened since your wife died?' *

Jack: 'Oh God no, it goes back 20 years. There was a big fuss, it was something to do with what we called our second child. We'd always loved the name Melanie, only to find that she was expecting a baby as well and she wanted to call it Melanie, and she felt we'd stolen her name—never forgiven us for it'.

Visitor: 'Well, that's a problem that's obviously been going on for a very long time, but can we come back to you and how you are feeling now, because it's—what—nearly 3 months since your wife died?'

In the above sequence the visitor, while acknowledging that Jack has a problem, is making it quite clear that that problem is not within her remit to work with.

By setting boundaries which are understood and agreed by both the worker and the bereaved person, there is less likelihood of misunderstandings creeping in, or for over-dependence or the need for friendship. Of course there are occasions when friendships do occur in any work setting. The bereavement visitor may see a number of grieving people throughout the year, and one or two of them may pull something from her in terms of emotion that the others do not, and from this it is possible that a life-long friendship may result. However, this should always been seen as the exception rather than the rule.

SUMMARY

In this chapter, some of the potential problems of bereavement visiting have been addressed:

- While accepting that those who have suffered the death of somebody that they loved are vulnerable, strategies have been explored to avoid dependency, transference and the developing of inappropriate friendships.
- It has also been noted that sometimes the people who work with the bereaved have unmet needs themselves which may be met by befriending the bereaved person. The dangers of this have been addressed.
- Finally, it has been suggested that boundaries on the purpose and function of bereavement visits should be set, not only by the bereavement visitor, but with the person that they are visiting.

REFERENCE

Faulkner A, Maguire P 1994 Talking to cancer patients and their families. Oxford University Press, Oxford

The cost of care

The cost of care is well documented (Maslach 1981, Faulkner & Maguire 1988, Burnard 1991, Faulkner 1992) but, as was seen in previous chapters, there are particular risks in working with bereaved people if limits and boundaries are not set, not only in terms of commitment to a particular individual, but also in terms of total case load.

SELF-AWARENESS

Working with the bereaved is seldom a full-time commitment. For example, Cruse counsellors give an agreed number of hours a week to counselling as a voluntary contribution in addition to their full-time job or other family commitments. Nurses in hospices or the community may see family members after a death as a follow-up to check how they are coping. The size of the case load at any particular time should be an individual decision based on knowledge of oneself and how much time and energy can be given to those who are struggling to cope with a profound life crisis.

Most people, if asked, would say that they knew themselves very well, and if pressed further would give some descriptors of their personality and their attitude to life. What many people are less likely to do is to understand why they get stressed in particular situations, why they react in a particular way to a particular person, or indeed to examine the 'luggage' that they bring with them to each new situation from their past life experiences. Many people would see such introspection as almost unhealthy rather than as an aid to setting realistic limits based on self-knowledge.

In fact, constant introspection is not required but what is useful is for an individual to ask themselves why, if they take on a

---

Box 11.1 A case of counter transference

Nurse Black was working in the community as a district nurse. She always followed up the significant members of a family after a death and if she felt they were in need would continue to see them over a contracted period of time. She had four bereaved people in her case load when she realized that she had a problem. All were elderly and had lost a partner.

Her problem lay with Mrs Denver who seemed to need more from her than the others. She found that, although she had contracted to see Mrs Denver once a fortnight, if she was passing she would drop in and just say hello to the old lady and stay for a few moments. Such extra visits were not planned but seemed to take place almost unconsciously. The old lady always made her very welcome and was usually prepared to ask her to have a cup of tea and chat about things far removed from the bereavement. It was only when Nurse Black realized that she sometimes diverted past the old lady's house unnecessarily that she talked her problem over with a confidante.

Nurse Black had been a lonely and sometimes unhappy child. She was one of a large family whose mother was always busy with the newest baby. As the elder daughter in the family she had had to do a good many chores and often wondered, when she was in bed at night, if her parents really loved her.

When she started school there was an elderly lady living a few doors away who would often be on the doorstep and would invite the little girl into her house for a glass of milk and to look at some of her treasures. With her mother's permission, this old lady had become a significant feature of the little girl's life and precious memories of her had been maintained for a very long time after the old lady had died.

In talking through her dilemma of the old lady who was bereaved, Nurse Black realized that she had in fact taken those feelings from her childhood and succumbed to the old lady's invitations to tea and chat in the same way that she had done as a child. This is called counter transference, where another person reminds one of someone they were fond of previously so that that person begins to fulfil the same needs that the remembered person did. Once Nurse Black gained insight, she was able to put this elderly lady into perspective in terms of responsibilities and contracting for visits. It caused both of them a little heartache but was dealt with before the feelings became too strong.

'difficult' case, they are experiencing problems. This will usually help to put the difficulties into perspective and to identify if they are related to past life experience.

Transference and counter transference

Counter transference can work the other way in that a client may remind the visitor of somebody that they do not like, and then they find that it is very difficult to warm to the particular bereaved person. With insight, no damage need be done, particularly if the bereavement visitor has the foresight to deal with the feelings or the opportunity to hand that particular case on to someone else.

Transference was explored in Chapter 10 in terms of the risk to the contracted relationship. What is also important to understand is that when transference occurs, counter transference may result. The positive side of counter transference is that by invoking feelings in the bereavement visitor, and if those feelings are examined and understood, it can give the visitor better insight into the feelings of the person who is bereaved.

Uncomfortable feelings

Such insight may lead to the realization that it is not always possible, for example, to be non-judgmental. The uncomfortable feelings may result from coming into contact with a lifestyle that is very different from one's own and which may in fact be unacceptable at a personal level. In giving some thought to the responses that are invoked by a bereaved person, it is possible to learn more about oneself and perhaps grow, so that it is possible in future encounters to be truly more non-judgmental than before.

In most situations it is not necessary to give up working with a bereaved person because of the feelings they invoke, but if it is necessary because the feelings are strong enough to begin to cause stress, then it is important that the changeover from one visitor to another should be made with the informed consent of the bereaved person concerned. A comfort here is the fact that if strong feelings are invoked in the bereavement visitor, it is highly likely that similar feelings are invoked in the bereaved person.

RESPONSIBILITIES

Most health professionals are trained and educated to believe that their role in life is to cure whatever problem the patient or family member may have, be it physical, psychological or social. In working with dying patients and their families, both before and after death, the realization comes that this is an area where problems must be resolved if possible by the individual concerned. This raises the issue of responsibility. Too often, those who work with the bereaved take on the responsibility for that person working through their grief and coming out at the other end open to new relationships.

A facilitator

Worden (1992) gives a useful paradigm in that he puts the responsibility for working through grief clearly with the bereaved person. This means that those who work with bereaved people have the role of facilitator rather than problem solver. By accepting that this is the case, the bereavement visitor is less likely to feel guilty or have a sense of failure when the bereaved person involved does not move on as fast as they should.

Certainly it is rewarding to see people move on through their grief, but in terms of personal survival in this area of work, it is necessary to accept that there will be people who are locked in their grief and may only recover with more expert help than a bereavement visitor can offer.

BALANCE

The key to personal survival when one is working with bereaved people is to maintain some sense of balance. This is why it is so important to recognize when a particular individual begins to take up more time than they should for their bereavement visits, and also why it is so important to contract and set limits at the outset of any involvement with a bereaved person.

Stress levels

This balance is not always easy to attain. If the bereavement work, for example, is voluntary following a full-time job and there is a family at home waiting to be fed, then stress levels may rise. A certain level of stress can be very stimulating and enhance day to day events. The difficulty is in recognizing when stress levels get out of hand. Meichenbaum (1983) puts stress into perspective by commenting that it is not something out there waiting to make your life a misery, it is what happens when you and the environment interact. It may also be seen as a warning that the current case load is more than can be managed comfortably while keeping the rest of life in balance.

Burn out

Signs that balance is not being maintained in life come on slowly and subtly. It may be that tempers begin to get frayed, that there is a tiredness that was not felt before. These signs should not be ignored, for they may be the first signs of burn out (Burnard 1991).

Reducing the case load

If stress levels rise it is important to take time to consider what is different in day to day work. It may be, for example, that a bereaved person is being particularly demanding, or it may be that the current case load includes particularly heart-breaking stories. When such feelings occur, it is worth considering reducing the case load or changing some aspect of life to bring matters back into balance.

Too often, committed health professionals work long hours so that the pleasure of going home and cooking a meal becomes a chore, or the thought of going out in the evening is just too much. It is at times like this that friends and family members can be most supportive by pointing out what has happened.

SUPERVISION

Supervision can be an important factor in maintaining balance, both in terms of case load, the type of case, and the mix of individuals with which one works. Unfortunately this is not available to all who work with bereaved people. If it is not available then it is of paramount importance that the individual carer finds someone who they can talk to on a regular basis about the cases that they are dealing with.

Without this facility it is very easy to become overloaded and tense and unable to share problems which, if not discussed, can become out of proportion.

A trusted colleague

The need to talk to a supervisor or a trusted colleague can be particularly important when there is a difficult case to deal with. It may be, for example, that the bereaved person has a very difficult history with a death that caused them large problems. Or it may be that the bereavement visitor finds it particularly difficult to tune in to this person and their problems. In order to survive in this difficult area, it is necessary to switch off those feelings so that one can go on to the next task or go home at the end of a working day. Again, insight should be attempted, for rather than feeling low and fed-up, it helps to ask the question,

'Why do I feel so low and fed-up?' and then the answer may be,

'because of the particular feelings invoked by somebody's story'.

LETTING GO

Working with bereaved people can be very rewarding in that their movement from utter desolation to seeing a future where they can be happy again may reinforce a sense of purpose and attainment. The difficult part is in letting that person go to continue their movement towards new relationships on their own. By contracting and reviewing, this letting go should be more manageable but again, with insight, it can often be seen that where the bereavement visitor is meeting the needs of an individual, working with that individual may well be meeting needs within the bereavement visitor.

It is not uncommon for a bereaved person to be seeing a visitor or counsellor many years after a death. This is particularly true where the bereavement service offers some sort of social function and, rather than coming for a few months and then moving on to other things, the person continues to use the social gathering as their only interaction with groups of other people. Only by understanding our own feelings are we able to let go. A rule of thumb is that all contracts need to be regularly reviewed, not only in terms of how the bereaved person is progressing, but also in terms of whether this contract is changing to meet needs in the bereavement visitor.

SUMMARY

In this brief chapter, some of the particular aspects of working with bereaved people have been considered in terms of the cost of this work to those who are involved. These include:

- setting personal limits based on knowledge of self and on how much one can be involved in this area of work
- the need to leave responsibility for recovery from loss to the bereaved individual along with the need to maintain a sense of balance between work and play the role of supervision has been briefly mentioned along with the need to talk through problem areas
- finally, the hardest task of all has been noted, that of letting go when the bereaved individual is showing signs of moving on from their grief towards recovery.

The references cited in this chapter provide further reading on the cost of care and the need for support for those who work in health care.

REFERENCES

Burnard P 1991 Beyond burn out. Nursing Standard 5 (43):46–48
Faulkner A, Maguire P 1988 The need for support. Nursing 5 (28): 1010–1012
Maslach C 1981 Burn out—the cost of caring. Prentice Hall, New Jersey
Meichenbaum D 1983 Coping with stress. Multi Media Publications (UK) Ltd

Summary of responsibilities and boundaries

In the absence of clear guidelines bereavement visits may be no more than 'tea and sympathy' and those relatives at risk of abnormal grief may be missed by those who have not been taught to distinguish between normal and abnormal grief.

The purpose of a bereavement visit is to assess:

1. whether grieving has commenced
2. whether the grief is within normal limits
3. whether there is any sign, no matter how small, that adaptation has commenced.

Timing is important, for the first week or so may seem almost unreal, but 6 weeks or so after the death the bereaved person should be on a slope towards adaptation to the loss.

THE BEREAVEMENT VISIT

Negotiation

Negotiate over timing of visit, so that you are expected, rather than turning up on the doorstep without warning.

Introduction

Remind the bereaved person of the purpose of the visit, e.g.

'I understand that you were wanting to talk to someone. I'd like to begin by asking you about John's death. Are you sure it's OK with you?'

Encourage precision

It is important to gain an accurate perspective from the bereaved person. This also fulfills the function of putting them in touch with their feelings, e.g.

'It is 6 weeks now since John died. Can you tell me exactly how it was for you?' rather than,

'Can you tell me about your sad loss?'

Other questions should include:

- When exactly did John die?
- What time?
- Were you there? (If not, how did you find out? Were you alone? What did you do?)
- How did John die?
- Can you tell me exactly what happened?
- Were you alone—or was support available?

Explore feelings

Be prepared to explore and encourage the expression of feelings without being voyeuristic. The aim is to allow the articulation of those events which society encourages bereaved individuals to suppress.

If the bereaved person was present at death explore both feelings and reactions, e.g.

- 'You say he made a horrible noise—how did that leave you feeling?'
- 'So there was blood dribbling from her mouth. How did you feel when you saw that?'

At this point you will need to note any signs of non-acceptance, e.g.

- 'It didn't seem real'.
- 'It was like seeing someone else'.
- 'Like watching a film'.

If this type of statement is made, it is important to check if things have changed, e.g.

* 'You say it didn't seem real—how long did that last?'

If the bereaved person was not present at death, it is important to explore why, e.g.

* 'If I'd only known I would have been there' versus
* 'I couldn't stay—it was so awful—he had wasted away'.

Feelings about this may include anger due to misinformation and/or guilt at having 'failed' a loved one. Those who had made a rational decision not to be there may or may not regret it, or react badly in retrospect.

If the bereaved individual was not present, did she see the body after death? How did she feel. Again, you are looking for signs of non-acceptance, and any subsequent change.

Death—funeral

You need to gain as precise an account as possible of the sequence of events covering the time from death through to the funeral. What type of service—burial or cremation? Were they involved in the arrangements? Did they attend? Were other family members supportive?

This may well be a difficult area for a bereaved person to describe. You should encourage disclosure while respecting the person's pain, e.g.

Visitor: 'You say it seemed unreal when you saw Colin. How were you by the time of the funeral?'

Joan: 'I managed—I had to. He wanted cremation–no one else would have made sure it was how he wanted it'.

Clarifying feelings

You need to establish the nature, frequency and intensity of feelings after the initial period of shock or numbness, e.g.

* 'You say you managed well during the time of the funeral but were you able to show your feelings?'
* 'In what way?'

- 'When did that start?'

This will help you assess:

1. If feelings were expressed or suppressed.
2. If feelings are tolerable or overwhelming—'I felt I was losing control—going mad'.
3. The level of pre-occupation with thoughts of the dead person during waking and sleeping time.
   'He seems always there. At night I dream of him being fun, loving, whispering the silly lovely things—like the way he would say "Good morning" meaning "it's good with you"—and then the day is bad because I miss him like I didn't think was possible'.
4. If searching behaviour has occurred,
   'I find myself outside his office—often I can't remember walking there' or,
   'I go to the Hospice—walk around the garden where we used to sit—they must think I'm mad'.
5. If hallucinations have occurred, their frequency and intensity,
   'I was going shopping and I found myself waiting outside the gate. She was there—I believe now in spirits—it's sort of comforting in a way, knowing she hasn't gone completely'.

Present feelings

At the time of assessment you are looking for change in level of feelings from those of the first 2–3 weeks. You might say 'it has obviously been a very difficult time for you—tell me, how different it is now?' Remember to check nature, intensity and duration of feelings and to acknowledge that change can be in either direction. Any of the following patterns may emerge.

Downward slope (resolving)

'It still hurts like hell, but I laughed the other day and for a moment felt almost happy'.

Upward slope (accelerating)

'It's worse. At first I could think of other things but now its round and round. . . . ! '

Box 12.1   Grief not appropriate

Note   It is important to clarify whether grief is appropriate when it is absent e.g. if dead relative was mean, unpleasant and unloved, and his death means the possibility of the Porsche from his inheritance, grieving is unlikely and its absence no problem.

Feelings remain intense (chronic grief)

'It hasn't changed at all—I wonder if it ever will?'

Remains unable to express grief (absent grief)

'It's under control—I can't give in to it'.

Begins to express grief, but represses, then starts . . . . .
(oscillating grief)

'It was too painful—I couldn't stop crying so I put the lid on . . . . then something happens and I start again . . . I have to keep it in as much as I can'.

Acceptance of death

There are key questions which will help you assess if the relative has accepted the death.

'Are you able to visit the grave/crematorium?'

The reply will indicate one of the following situations:

1. Normal pattern emerging
2. Total avoidance (reason?)
3. Visits too often (reason?).

Box 12.2   Exploding grief

Note   The danger with both absent and oscillating grief is that a 'trigger' may lead to exploding grief which needs immediate specialist help.

'How do you feel when you do visit?'

Responses will vary and may amplify pattern of visiting.

1. 'It helps me to go—sort of comforting—taking flowers—feeling I'm a bit nearer'.
2. 'It's just too painful—I just get to the gate—its all there—sorry . . . . .'.
3. 'I get horrible feelings—I know she is in there—I want to get her out—last time—I just had to run'.
4. 'When I get there I don't want to leave. I find myself talking to him. Yesterday I took my little tape-recorder—playing Streisand—you know—I don't know what other people thought'.

'What about Jack's things?'

If some things were given away, what has been kept? Were they given away in haste or still around as if he were there? Again, reactions vary.

1. 'I took his clothes and things to Oxfam—only last week—but I've kept his decanters on the dresser—and his trophies—I don't want to forget him'.
2. 'It's all as it was—just waiting for him. I don't let anyone in'.
3. 'I've hidden them—it's all too much'.
4. 'It's the photographs I can't bear to see—perhaps one day'.

'What sort of memories do you have of John?'

Memories may be very negative, suppressed, or they may begin to be able to connect with positive ones.

1. 'I see him in the hospital, in pain, and I wish I could shut him out'.
2. 'I try not to think, I'm trying to move on. It's over—finished'.
3. 'It's getting easier—my father took me out for dinner the other night—the last time in that restaurant was with John—suddenly I remembered that night—how he dealt so smoothly with the staff and how special I felt about him. We had a silly quarrel but suddenly it was all right—he gave me one of those looks and I melted. Is it wrong to remember lovely things when I should be sad?'

Other questions

Other questions will show you if the person is remembered in the past or kept in the present (this may link in with the room kept ready). If death was sudden with no body, as in a disaster, there may be no real acceptance of the death.

Blocking factors

If a bereaved person seems to be blocking, you need to explore relevant factors. This needs to be done very sensitively.

How they feel now

It is useful to ask how the individual feels about dead person now. This can sometimes elicit feelings of anger, guilt or irritation which should be explored.

Other problems

Screen for other problems.

Support in the family

Ask about support available in family/social circle.

Children

Any children? How have they coped?

The future

If the future hasn't been mentioned, ask about plans.

A further visit

Offer a further visit if you feel it necessary (see Decisions).

DECISIONS AND BOUNDARIES

After the assessment you should decide:

1. Is grief pattern normal, i.e. are feelings less intensive now than when grieving started? Can the individual talk about the dead person, using his name? Is she sorting out/giving away possessions, keeping cherished mementos? Is he visiting grave in balanced way? Is she thinking about the future?

2. Is the grief pattern abnormal, i.e. are feelings as intense, more intense, oscillating, or absent? Is the relative unable to mention the patient's name? Unreasonably angry with him for dying? Over-guilty for things left undone? Are possessions unmoved? Is there a shrine? Were possessions given away with undue haste? Is the grave visited too often? Not at all? Does the future look bleak? Are there symptoms of clinical depression?

Box 12.3 Be alert

Note Although one expects to see a downward slope in two months, it must be remembered that individuals do vary; but be alert if grief seems entirely absent or too intense.

Box 12.4 Action options

1. No further reaction if satisfied grief within normal limits, but leave telephone number.
2. Further visit if you feel there is need for support and/or further assessment.
3. Refer to other agency if grief seems absent or outside normal limits.

The boundaries

If further visits seem necessary these should be clearly contracted, e.g.

'Would it help if I visited you again, then after the next 3 visits we will re-assess the situation'.

This may seem hard but the alternative, i.e. to go on visiting without contracting, can encourage dependency which is difficult to break.

FURTHER READING

Alexander H 1993 Bereavement: a shared experience. Lion Publishing, Oxford

Burnell G 1989 Clinical management of bereavement: a handbook of healthcare professionals. Human Sciences Press, New York

Clark D 1993 The sociology of death. Blackwell Scientific, Oxford

Dickenson D, Johnson M (eds) 1993 Death, dying and bereavement. Sage Publications, London

Dillenburger K 1992 Violent bereavement. Ashgate Publishing Group, Avebury

Duffy W 1991 The bereaved child: A guide for teachers and leaders. The National Society for Children, London

Faulkner A 1993 Developments in bereavement services. In: Clark D (ed.) The future for palliative care. Open University Press, London

Furman E 1981 A child's parent dies: studies in childhood bereavement. Yale University Press, Newhaven

Gersie A 1991 Storymaking in bereavement. Jessica Kingsley Publishers, London

Gorer G 1965 Death, grief and mourning. Cresset Press, London

Green J, Green M 1992 Dealing with death: practices and procedures. Chapman & Hall, London

Gunzburg J 1993 Unresolved grief. Chapman & Hall, London

Hill L 1994 Caring for dying children and their families. Chapman & Hall, London

Houlbrook R 1989 Death, ritual and bereavement. Routledge, London

Jones M 1988 Secret flowers. The Women's Press, London

Lewis C S 1966 A grief observed. Faber, London

Littlewood J 1992 Aspects of grief: bereavement in adult life. Routledge, London

Murgatroyd S, Woolfe R 1982 Coping with crisis. Open University Press, London. (Reprinted 1993)

Neuberger J 1987 Caring for dying people of different faiths. Austin Cornish/Lisa Sainsbury, London

Parkes C M, Weiss R S 1983 Recovery from bereavement. Tavistock Press, London

Penson J 1990 Bereavement: a guide for nurses. Harper & Row, London

Richardson R 1991 Talking about bereavement. Optima, London

Sanders C 1989 The mourning after: dealing with adult bereavement. John Wiley & Sons, Chichester

Sherr L 1989 Death, dying and bereavement: an insight for carers. Blackwell Scientific Publications, Glasgow

Sheskin A 1979 Cryonics: a sociology of death and bereavement. John Wiley & Sons, Chichester

Wallbank S 1991 Facing grief: bereavement and the young adult. Lutterworth Press, London

USEFUL ADDRESSES

National Association of Bereavement Services
20 Norton Folgate
LONDON
E1 6DB
Tel: 0171 247 1080

Bereavement Trust
Stamford Hall
LOUGHBOROUGH
Leics
Tel: 01509 852333

British Association of Health Services in Higher Education
Reading University Health Services
9 Northcourt Avenue
READING, Berks
Tel: 01734 874551

Civil Service Fellowship
1B Deals Gateway
Blackheath Road
LONDON SE10 8BW
Tel: 0181 691 7411

Foundation for the study of infant deaths (SIDS)
35 Belgrave Square
LONDON SW1X 8PS
Tel: 0171 235 1721/0965

National Association for Widows
54–57 Allison Street
Digbeth
BIRMINGHAM B5 5TH
Tel: 0121 643 8348

Shadow of Suicide (SOS)
109 Abbeyville Road
LONDON SW4 8JL
Tel: 0171 622 7932

Index

For my mother

'When a lovely flame dies,
Smoke gets in your eyes.'

Harback

For Churchill Livingstone:

Commissioning Editor: Ellen Green
Project Development Editor: Mairi McCubbin
Project Manager: Valerie Burgess
Project Controller: Pat Miller
Design Direction: Judith Wright
Indexer: Valerie Elliston

Working with Bereaved People